The Institute of Biology's
*Studies in Biology no. 36*

# Nervous Systems

by *Peter N. R. Usherwood*
B.Sc., Ph.D., M.I.Biol., F.R.S.E.

Senior Lecturer in Zoology
University of Glasgow

Edward Arnold

*First published 1973*
by Edward Arnold (Publishers) Limited,
25 Hill Street,
London, W1X 8LL


Boards edition  ISBN: 0 7131 2369 9
Paper edition    ISBN: 0 7131 2370 2

Printed in Great Britain by
The Camelot Press Ltd., London and Southampton

# General Preface to the Series

It is no longer possible for one textbook to cover the whole field of Biology and to remain sufficiently up to date. At the same time students at school, and indeed those in their first year at universities, must be contemporary in their biological outlook and know where the most important developments are taking place.

The Biological Education Committee, set up jointly by the Royal Society and the Institute of Biology, is sponsoring, therefore, the production of a series of booklets dealing with limited biological topics in which recent progress has been most rapid and important.

A feature of the series is that the booklets indicate as clearly as possible the methods that have been employed in elucidating the problems with which they deal. Wherever appropriate there are suggestions for practical work for the student. To ensure that each booklet is kept up to date, comments and questions about the contents may be sent to the author or the Institute.

1973                                        INSTITUTE OF BIOLOGY
                                            41 Queen's Gate
                                            London, S.W.7

# Preface

One outstanding major scientific goal is to discover how the human brain works. Unfortunately we are still a long way from achieving this ambition; indeed, we do not yet understand the nervous systems of simple animals which contain only a few hundred nerve cells, let alone that complex universe of some billions of nerve cells which comprises the human brain. However, the complexity of the problem engenders fascination and the very magnitude of the task makes the challenge all the more worth while.

It is my belief that progress in this field will be facilitated by studies of simple as well as complex nervous systems and I have therefore attempted, within the limitations of this booklet, to present a comparative account of the structure and function of vertebrate and invertebrate nervous systems. The approach is introductory rather than comprehensive and my only hope is that the information that I have presented will fire some of you with sufficient enthusiasm to enquire further into this exciting world.

Glasgow 1973                                        P. N. R. U.

# Contents

1 Introduction 1
  1.1 Structural properties of nerve cells 2
  1.2 Synapses 5
  1.3 Evolution of the nervous system 7

2 Nervous Organization 10
  2.1 Coelenterates 10
  2.2 Echinoderms 12
  2.3 Platyhelminthes 12
  2.4 Annelids 13
  2.5 Arthropods 13
  2.6 Molluscs 14
  2.7 Vertebrates 15
  2.8 The vertebrate brain 19
  2.9 Autonomic nervous systems 22

3 Excitable Properties of Nerve Cells 25
  3.1 Introductory electrochemistry 25
  3.2 Electrochemistry of neurons 32
  3.3 Resting membrane potential 36
  3.4 Generation of electrical signals 36
  3.5 The ionic basis of the action potential 38
  3.6 Passive electrical properties of neurons 40
  3.7 The action potential and nervous conduction 43
  3.8 Electrophysiological techniques 49

4 Synaptic Transmission 52
  4.1 Chemical synapses 52
  4.2 Electrical synapses 60
  4.3 Presynaptic inhibition 60

5 Sensory Receptors and Sense Organs 61
  5.1 General principles 61
  5.2 Mechanoreception 65
  5.3 Photoreception 79
  5.4 Optokinesis 86

6 Integrative Properties of Nervous Systems 88
  6.1 Integration at synapses 88
  6.2 Nerve nets 93
  6.3 Reflexes and nervous integration 96

7   Memory                                                    107
   7.1   Short-term memory in insects                    109
   7.2   Synapses and short-term memory                  111
   7.3   Long-term memory                                112
   7.4   DNA, RNA and memory                             112
   7.5   Synapses and long-term memory                   114
   7.6   Memory in mammals                               115

Books for Further Reading                                    117

References                                                   117

Index                                                        119

# Introduction

All living organisms respond to stimuli of one kind or another. We know from personal experience that live animals respond to many different forms of stimulation whereas dead animals and inanimate objects usually do not. Most human animals are distressed when confronted with a goldfish floating upside down in a fish tank or a rabbit lying immobile on its side on a country path and the more inquisitive amongst us would usually wish to determine whether these animals are alive or dead. We would do this by testing their irritability. We would touch (stimulus) the goldfish or rabbit to see if it moves (response).

Although all the cells of multicellular animals are irritable to some extent the reception of stimuli from the external and internal environments of these animals is usually the prerogative of specialized cells, the sensory cell or sensory receptors. Sometimes the sensory cells form either a part of or the whole of an organ called, appropriately, a sense organ. The human eye is an example of a complex sense organ. When there is an overt response of an organism following receipt of a stimulus this results from the activity of another class of specialized cells, the effector cells, which may be grouped to form tissues such as muscles and glands. In the more advanced multicellular animals, the sensory receptors may be located some considerable distance from the effectors. How then is the activity of a distant effector influenced by or triggered by information (stimuli) received by a sensory receptor? A system which transmits information efficiently and quickly over long distances is clearly essential. To meet this requirement, cells have been set aside, specialized and organized to act as channels of communication between the sensory receptors on the one hand and the effectors on the other hand. These cells comprise a nervous system.

It would be very incorrect, however, to consider a nervous system as nothing more than a communication network. For instance, nerve cells functioning as sensory receptors select information from the vast amount of stimuli impinging on the surface of an animal, and components within a nervous system often integrate the inputs from spatially distinct and maybe even functionally distinct sensory receptors. Many nervous systems also have a decision-making capacity whereby information may be either channelled along selected pathways to specific effectors or may be prevented from reaching the effectors. More advanced nervous systems may incorporate the property of long-term information storage (memory) coupled with the facility to retrieve specific information from their memory banks when it is required. Finally, certain components or constellations of nerve cells may spontaneously generate patterns of activity which contribute to the overall behaviour of the animal.

In an acellular (unicellular) animal such as a protozoan the entire surface membrane is probably sensitive to many different stimuli although in some protozoans certain parts of this membrane exhibit enhanced sensitivity to specific stimuli. There is some evidence that the physicochemical basis for reception and transmission of information in acellular animals is the same as for the nervous systems of multicellular animals, but the mode of transmission of information from either the cell surface membrane, or receptor organelles, to the effector system or effector organelles in these animals has not yet been fully elucidated.

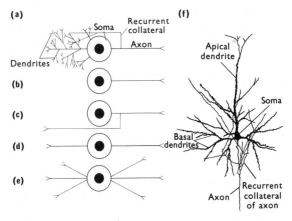

**Fig. 1–1** Neurons can be classified according to the number of processes which emerge from their somata. Some of the different types of neurons found in vertebrates and invertebrates are illustrated in (a–e). (a) A multipolar neuron with the facility for either self-excitation or self-inhibition through a recurrent axon pathway (vertebrate brain). (b) A monopolar neuron (arthropod motor neuron). (c) A branching monopolar neuron (vertebrate afferent neuron). (d) A bipolar neuron (coelenterate nerve net). (e) A multipolar neuron. (f) A drawing of a multipolar pyramidal neuron found in the sensori-motor cortex of a cat. Note the recurrent collateral of the axon which in this case is inhibitory and therefore provides for a negative feedback pathway onto the dendrites of the neuron. The dendrites are covered with spines which provide numerous sites for synapses between the dendrites and the collateral axon process and processes from other neurons. ( (e) is after SHOLL, 1956.)

## 1.1 Structural properties of nerve cells

A nervous system is a tissue and like all tissues is made up of units or cells (Plate 1). Since the nerve cell is usually quite distinct structurally from most other animal cells it is given a special name, i.e. it is called a neuron(e). Although neurons exhibit many diverse forms (Fig. 1–1), they have certain features in common. For example, each contains a nucleus which lies in an expanded part of the cell called the soma (perikaryon, cell body) (Fig. 1–2).

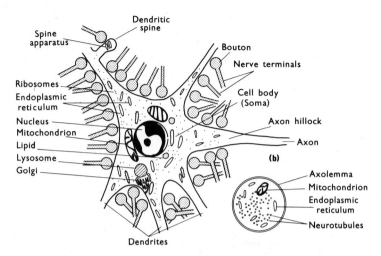

(a)

**Fig. 1–2** (a) Schematic representation of the soma region of a neuron. Dendrites, soma and axon make synaptic contact with endings (boutons) from other neurons. The axon is also shown diagrammatically in transverse section (b) to illustrate the presence of neurotubules, mitochondria and smooth endoplasmic reticulum. The membrane at the axon hillock region often has the lowest threshold for the production of action potentials. In some neurons, action potentials are generated by the soma membrane and possibly also by dendritic membrane but in other neurons these regions are electrically inexcitable. The relative distribution of synapses and action potential generating membranes in a neuron plays an important role in the functioning of the nerve cell. (Redrawn after BULLOCK & HORRIDGE, 1965.)

Two types of cell process or cytoplasm-filled tubes, called axons and dendrites, may arise from the soma. The axon (nerve fibre) is usually smooth and rarely branches except at its termination whereas the dendrites are frequently profusely branched. Neurons of lower invertebrates usually have a number of axonal processes and for this reason they are called multipolar neurons. Vertebrate neurons and neurons of higher invertebrates usually have only one axon although some neurons, such as the amacrine cells found in the human eye, lack a demonstrable axon altogether. Most vertebrate neurons are, nevertheless, multipolar since they have many dendritic processes.

When the neuron is viewed with the electron-microscope, it appears to be bounded by a membrane about 7·5 nm thick. It is unfortunate that there is much uncertainty about the nature of this membrane because knowledge of its molecular structure would be of great importance as a key to understanding the physicochemical basis for transmission of information in nerve cells since the membrane is greatly involved in this transmission process (*see* Section 3).

As yet there is little functional significance that can be attached to some of the structures occurring within neurons. The neurotubules which are found in all processes of the nerve cell may form continuous pipelines from the soma to the axon terminals and dendritic endings for transporting materials such as neurotransmitters and neurohormones. However, the cytoplasm of the nerve cell is continuously in motion and presumably also carries many important substances up and down the axons and dendrites.

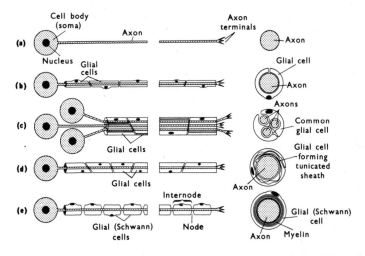

**Fig. 1–3** Diagrammatic representation of the types of relationship to be found between neurons and glial cells in the peripheral nervous systems of vertebrates and invertebrates. A row of glial cells invests either a single axon (b) or a group of axons (c). These arrangements are found in vertebrate and invertebrate nerves. The axon in (d) is invested by a row of glial cells each of which 'spins' a series of loose wrappings around the fibre to produce a tunicated sheath. This arrangement is characteristic of arthropod nerves. The vertebrate myelinated axon is illustrated in (e). Here the axon is enveloped by a sheath formed by spirally arranged membrane processes of glial (Schwann) cells which are very tightly packed. The naked axon in (a) is found in some coelenterate nervous systems.

In most animals the somata, axons and dendrites of nerve cells are surrounded by non-nervous cells called glial cells, which may contribute to complex sheath-like structures (Fig. 1–3). In most multicellular animals the peripheral axons with their associated glial cells are frequently grouped together and invested by a common connective tissue sheath to form a compound structure called a nerve. In insect and crustacean nerves the axons are invested by a loose sheath formed by wrappings of glial cell membranes but with cytoplasm between the membranes. These axons are said to be tunicated. The most common type of axonal sheath in vertebrate nerves is the myelin sheath. In this case the membranous processes of glial cells (Schwann cells) form a spiral around the axon and are packed so tightly that there is no cytoplasm between the wrappings (Plates 2, 3). A single Schwann cell provides the wrapping for about 2 mm of axon. The Schwann cells do not form a continuous sheath. In the gap, called the node of Ranvier, between two Schwann cells the axon membrane is exposed. The region between two nodes is called an internode. Axons with this type of sheath are described as myelinated (medullated), and we shall discover later that the myelin sheath has important consequences for the way in which information is conducted along such axons.

## 1.2 Synapses

The neuron is a highly specialized cell that has greatly developed properties of irritability and conductivity. Like other cells neurons are generally discrete entities and as such are separated from each other and from non-nervous cells by cell membranes. However, functional contacts between nerve cells do occur. Indeed, bridges of some type for transmission of information from one cell to the next are essential if communication throughout the nervous system is to be achieved. At one time it was considered likely that a neuron made protoplasmic contact with its neighbours. This reticular theory of nervous organization has now been largely superseded by the neuron theory which proposes that functional connections between individual nerve cells are effected by close contacts and not by continuity in a syncytial network (Plates 4 and 5). The term synapse has been applied to the region of contact or contiguity between two neurons, between a sensory receptor and a neuron, and between a neuron and an effector.

At synapses, information from a neuron or sensory receptor cell, the presynaptic element is transferred to another cell, i.e. either a second neuron or an effector cell, the postsynaptic element (Fig. 1–4). Neurons make synaptic contact with each other in a variety of ways. For example, synapses occur between axons (axo-axonal synapses), axons and somata (axo-somatic synapses) and axons and dendrites (axo-dendritic synapses). Neurons with profusely branched dendritic processes, such as the pyramidal cells found in the cerebral cortex of mammalian brains (Fig. 1.1(f)), can make contact with hundreds or even thousands of other neurons and this has important implications for the functioning of such cells and indeed for the functioning of the nervous system as a whole.

The gross and fine structural properties of synapses have received considerable attention from histologists and electron-microscopists. It is now agreed that the gross structure of a synapse depends on its mode of information transfer, or transmission. Some synapses transmit electrically and these are sometimes termed ephapses or tight junctions to distinguish them from the majority of synapses which transmit chemically. At both types of

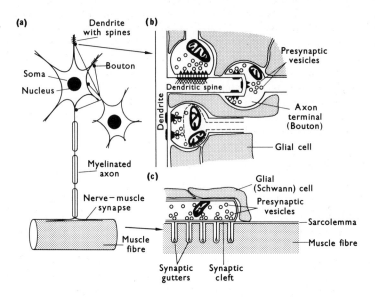

**Fig. 1-4** Diagrammatic representation of synapses between neurons, and between neurons and muscle fibres. (a) The axon of a motor neuron makes synaptic contact with a muscle fibre. This type of synapse is frequently called an end-plate. The terminal of the motor neuron contains mitochondria and synaptic vesicles. The membrane of the muscle fibre which lies under the axon terminal, i.e. the postsynaptic membrane, is folded (c). The motor neuron also synapses with another neuron (a). The synapses between these two neurons are mainly on the dendrites of the motor neuron but may also occur on the soma and axon (especially in the region of the axon hillock) of the motor neuron. The terminals of the presynaptic neuron contain mitochondria and synaptic vesicles (b). Other structures such as the postsynaptic web (top synapse in (b), the spine apparatus and the presynaptic projections (b), etc. may also be present although their roles are, at present, obscure.

synapse the membranes of the presynaptic and postsynaptic cells are separated by a cleft, the synaptic cleft (gap). Electrically-transmitting synapses are characterized by very narrow synaptic clefts, i.e. less than 10 nm in width, filled with dense material of unknown composition. Somewhat more diffuse material is found in clefts of most chemical synapses, the clefts being as narrow as 15 nm at some and as wide as 60 nm at others. Vesicles, 30–50 nm in diameter, perhaps appropriately called synaptic vesicles, are invariably found in the terminals of the presynaptic element at chemical synapses (Fig. 1-4). These vesicles are considered to contain the chemical (transmitter, transmitter substance, transmitter agent, neurotransmitter) used for transferring information across the synaptic cleft. Frequently, but not invariably, the synaptic vesicles are clustered opposite the synaptic cleft (Plate 5). The membrane which borders the presynaptic side of the synaptic cleft will be referred to as the presynaptic membrane. Although this membrane is responsible for releasing the chemical mediator from the presynaptic neuron during synaptic transmission, it is not obviously structurally differentiated from the rest of the surface membrane of this cell. That part of the membrane of the post-synaptic element, which is functionally specialized to recognize and transduce the information received in chemical form from the pre-synaptic cell, will be referred to as the postsynaptic membrane. However, this membrane appears very similar in fine structure to the rest of the membrane of the postsynaptic cell, although granules lining the outer face of the postsynaptic membrane have been seen in some electron micrographs. The postsynaptic membrane of some vertebrate nerve-striated muscle synapses is greatly folded (Fig. 1–4(c)), the folds probably serving to increase the area of the receptive surface for the chemical released from the terminals of the presynaptic neuron.

Synaptic vesicles are infrequently found at electrically-transmitting synapses where they may occur presynaptically as well as postsynaptically. Their presence here seems rather anomalous, although it is important to bear in mind that many different forms of information may be transferred at synapses between cells. It is possible that trophic information is transmitted at these electrical synapses by secretion of chemicals stored in the 'synaptic vesicles'. There is also an intimate relationship between the nervous system and the endocrine system of an animal. Indeed special neurons called neuro-secretory neurons, which store and release neurohormones, are found in vertebrates and invertebrates, the neurohormones being stored in vesicles, like synaptic vesicles.

## 1.3 Evolution of the nervous system

We have seen that in an acellular animal the entire organism appears to function as a combined sensory receptor and effector (although spatial separation of receptor and effector function may occur, together with structural differentiation of effector and receptor organelles) but in multi-cellular animals sensory reception and motor function are the prerogative of specialized cells or groups of cells. Epithelial sensori-motor cells, in which the functions of sensory reception and motor activity are both represented, are found in simple multicellular animals such as coelenterates, although the receptor and effector organelles within these cells are always clearly demarcated. Possibly this was the primitive situation in the Metazoa before a true nervous system containing discrete nerve cells appeared (Fig. 1–5). The next step in the evolution of the nervous system possibly involved the separation of the receptor and effector components of these sensori-motor epithelial cells into discrete sensory and motor units. The sensory receptor cell may have initially maintained its connections with the effector cell by means of fine processes, but this mode of communication was possibly superseded by the interposition of other cells between the effectors and sensory receptors. Perhaps these intermediary cells also arose from epithelial cells which migrated inwards from the ectoderm and subsequently lost their sensori-motor properties to become structurally and functionally differentiated as the first nerve cells. By incorporating further nerve cells into this system to act as channels of communication between these intermediary cells, a simple nerve net of the type found in some coelenterates would have been created.

Although a simple nerve net provides an animal with a system for communication between its body parts, the mode of conduction of information within this type of nervous system is rather diffuse and somewhat localized. However, the development of preferred pathways of conduction

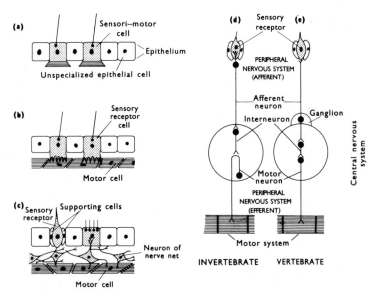

**Fig. 1–5** A hypothetical representation of the evolution of the nervous system. (a) The primitive sensori-motor system. (b) Separation of sensory and motor functions. (c) Interposition of a conduction system of neurons between sensory and motor cells to produce a nerve net of the type characterized by some coelenterate nervous systems. (d) Development of a central nervous system and appearance of central interneurons to produce an organization which is characteristic of the invertebrate nervous system where the somata of interneurons and motor neurons are arranged peripherally within the central nervous system. (e) The generalized vertebrate nervous system with somata of interneurons and motor neurons occupying a central position within the nerve cord.

whereby information could be 'directed' to certain sites, possibly along high-speed channels, would have overcome these restrictions and this may have been one major advance in the development of the nervous system. The next evolutionary step may have resulted in the aggregation of neurons into ganglia. This may have foreshadowed the appearance of the central nervous system, which is characteristic of higher metazoans, where neurons with specific functions in common are often concentrated and linked by special tracts of communication.

The general increase in boldily size, that has occurred during evolution and that has accompanied the development of a true central nervous system, has often resulted in a marked spatial separation of central neurons from effectors and sensory receptors. This problem has been solved by the development of neurons with long processes. Afferent (sensory) axons (fibres) connect receptors with the central nervous system on the one hand while efferent sensory (motor) axons connect central neurons with the effectors on the other hand. The afferent and efferent axons are often contained in nerves and, in those animals which possess a central nervous system, these nerves together with the sensory receptors constitute the peripheral nervous system. Other neurons, which are interpolated between the afferent and efferent cells, are called interneurons (intermediate neurons, intercalated neurons, internuncial neurons).

Before proceeding with a brief comparative description of nervous systems found in the animal kingdom it would perhaps be relevant to draw attention to one important aspect of nervous evolution. It will be seen that the nervous system has become specialized during the ascent from the lower metazoans to man. It is quite true that structural complexity of the neuron increases to some extent as the nervous system becomes more complex but we must not allow this to blind us to the fact that the building blocks of the nervous system are basically the same throughout the entire animal kingdom and that a coelenterate neuron is essentially similar in structure and function to a human nerve cell. Nervous complexity has been achieved not by drastically altering neurons, but by multiplying their numbers and by increasing their interconnections.

# Nervous Organization 2

By studying and comparing the nervous systems of animals from different phyla, it is possible to build up some sort of picture of the evolutionary development of the nervous system from a 'simple' network of neurons to the highly complex nervous organization found in man. However, it is important to remember that the level of nervous organization in any particular animal is intimately bound up with the mode of life of that animal so that sessile and parasitic forms of even advanced phyla might well be expected to exhibit a relatively low grade of nervous organization.

## 2.1 Coelenterates

Amongst contemporary free-living animals, the simplest nervous systems are found in the coelenterates (e.g. jellyfish, sea anemones, corals). In these animals the nerve net is the most prominent characteristic of the nervous system. This is best seen in its simplest form in some of the less mobile coelenterates, like *Hydra*, where it is chiefly sub-epidermal and consists of bipolar or tripolar neurons. These either fuse to form a syncytium without synapses or form non-polarized synapses capable of transmitting information in chemical form in both directions across the synaptic clefts. A somewhat higher grade of nervous organization is found in some other coelenterates especially in some of the motile forms. For example, in the ephyra larva of the jellyfish *Aurelia* there are two nerve nets with different structural and functional characteristics. One of these is very much like the diffuse nerve net of *Hydra* while the other conducts information in a much more undirectional or polarized manner, often at considerable speeds compared with the diffuse net. The latter is called a through-conduction net. However, the diffuse net and the through-conduction net both consist of discrete neurons, which communicate with each other and with receptor cells and effectors via synapses. Sometimes it is difficult to distinguish

Fig. 2-1 (a)   Diagram of the common jellyfish, *Aurelia*, showing position of rhopalia at the ends of each perradial and interradial canal. These structures are important sensory centres and are also responsible for initiating and co-ordinating the rhythmic swimming movements of this coelenterate. (After SHIPLEY & MACBRIDE, 1920.) (b) Hypothetical organization of a jellyfish ganglion (rhopalium) showing the three main nervous structures that have so far been distinguished. These consist of sensory cells and neurons which connect up with two nerve nets, a diffuse or 'slow' net and a 'fast' through-conduction net. (From *Interneurons: their Origin, Action, Specificity, Growth, and Plasticity* by G. ADRIAN HORRIDGE. W. H. Freeman and Company. Copyright © 1968.)

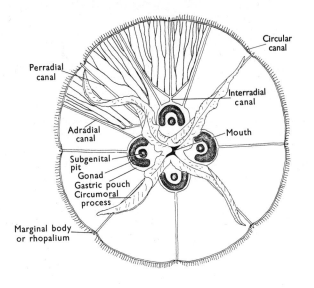

(a)

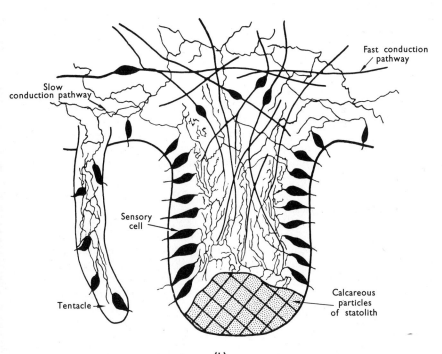

(b)

between a system such as this, with its two clearly defined networks of neurons and a system such as is found in, for example, sea anemones, in which a single nerve net contains both diffusely-conducting and through-conducting components. Sometimes the diffuse nets and through-conduction nets are called, respectively, 'slow' and 'fast' nets.

The development of the nervous system in the coelenterates reaches its peak in some of the free-swimming medusae with the formation of local concentrations of nerve cells (ganglia) and the appearance of tracts of nerve fibres, the so-called nerve rings. It is possible that the nerve rings foreshadow the nerves of higher animals although it would be incorrect to call them nerves since they are not distinctly demarcated from the adjacent tissues. In the common jellyfish there are eight ganglia distributed around the margin of the bell and these are connected by two nerve rings, which run round the margin of the bell. The ganglia, which are found at the end of each adradial and perradial canals, are called rhopalia (marginal bodies, tentaculocysts) and are important sensory centres for mechanoreception and photoreception (Fig. 2–1(a)). The ganglionic neurons send processes into the two nerve rings and also communicate with the nerve nets of the subumbrella and superumbrella surfaces of the bell (Fig. 2–1(b)).

## 2.2 Echinoderms

The nervous system of echinoderms approaches that of coelenterates, although there is slightly greater centralization. In the starfish, for example, there is a nerve ring around the mouth, called the oral ring, and five radial nerve tracks, one for each arm. The radial nerves communicate with a peripheral nerve plexus which innervates the muscles and sense organs of the arms. The nerve plexus is differentiated morphologically and function-ally into a 'fast' through-conduction system and a 'slow' diffuse conduction system. Possibly this plexus is equivalent to a nerve net although there is no doubt that direction of information along specific pathways is more pro-nounced in the echinoderm nervous system than it is in the coelenterate nervous system.

## 2.3 Platyhelminthes

Although it is debatable whether the starfish has a true central nervous system there is little doubt that such a structure is found in some of the free-living platyhelminthes. The fact that this centralization of nervous organization has been accompanied by the appearance of bilateral sym-metry is not at all coincidental. With the development of head to tail orientation many major sensory structures are found in the head since it is this region of the body which first samples the new environment during forward locomotion. Concentration of sensory receptors on the head has led to an equivalent concentration of neurons in this region to form a ganglionic mass or primitive brain. Even in these lowly animals this probably not only acts as an area for reception and integration of signals for the head receptors, but also receives information from sensory structures in other parts of the body and directs and controls the behaviour of many effectors. The central nervous system of flatworms like *Planaria* consists of one or more longitudinal nerve cords as well as a brain. Processes from neurons in the flatworm central nervous system pass out along nerves to make contact with a peripheral nerve plexus, which is associated with the musculature. This plexus is not a diffusely-conducting system and is not, therefore, equivalent to a nerve net. In the platyhelminth central nervous system the somata are separated from the main mass of axons and occupy a peripheral position in the ganglia and nerve cords, while the axons occupy a central position, where they form a neuro-pile. The central neurons are usually monopolar and the synaptic connections between neurons in the central nervous system occur almost exclusively in the neuropile, an arrangement which is generally characteristic of central nervous systems in invertebrates (Fig. 1–5(d)).

## 2.4  Annelids

In the annelids there is a clear-cut division of the nervous system into central and peripheral components. A distinct brain is usually present and in the higher annelids this may have fore, mid and hind regions. The brain is dorsal in position and is joined by connectives, which run around the gut, to a ventral nerve cord. The ventral nerve cord consists of paired, segmentally-arranged ganglia joined by paired connectives, although in some annelids lateral fusion of connectives and ganglia sometimes obscures their paired nature. Nerves containing both sensory and motor axons (i.e. mixed nerves) arise from the brain and segmental ganglia. These innervate the sensory and motor systems and also communicate with peripheral nerve plexuses found under the epidermis.

## 2.5  Arthropods

The general plan of the arthropod central nervous system consists of a well developed dorsal anterior brain (Fig. 2–2) with circumoesophageal connectives and a ventral nerve cord of segmental ganglia. The ganglia are, in reality, double structures, but this is not immediately obvious in some of the more advanced arthropods due to lateral fusion. The segmental arrangement of the ventral ganglia is also lost in some arthropods due to antero-posterior fusion of the ganglia and in extreme cases, such as in some species of fly, only one or, at the most, two ganglionic masses remain (Fig. 2–3). A useful indication of the sort of variation in the number and arrangement of the segmental ganglia in insects can be obtained by comparing the central nervous system of a cockroach or locust, where the

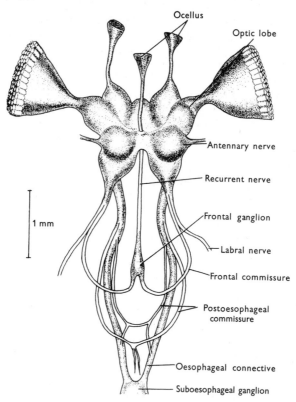

**Fig. 2–2** Anterior view of the brain of *Locusta migratoria*. Note that much of the brain is associated with the large sensory structures such as eyes and antennae found on the head of this insect. (After ALBRECHT, 1953.)

segmental nature of the ganglia is obvious with that of a housefly, where ganglion fusion is pronounced. One important feature of the somatic nervous system of arthropods is the absence of either nerve nets or nerve plexuses, although a nerve plexus may be associated with the visceral musculature. In this respect arthropods are similar to vertebrates.

## 2.6 Molluscs

The molluscan nervous system is as interesting as it is variable. Basically it consists of a series of paired ganglia, usually three or more, either connected by nerve tracts or fused to form a complex brain mass. In its simplest form the mollusc nervous system appears no better developed than that of a platyhelminth but in its most complex form as seen, for example, in the octopus the level of nervous organization compares

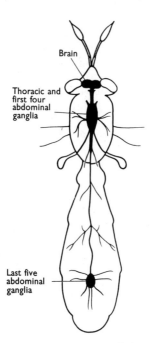

**Fig. 2-3**   Nervous system of a fly, *Physocephala*, showing distribution of very condensed ganglia of the ventral nerve cord. Only a few of the peripheral nerves are illustrated. (From SÉGUY, 1951.)

favourably with that of some lower vertebrates. Sub-epidermal plexuses which may mediate local reflexes not involving the central nervous system are found in many molluscs. For example, movements of a snail's foot are controlled, in part, by nervous activity patterns generated within a sub-epidermal nerve plexus.

Some of the most active predaceous invertebrate animals are to be found amongst the cephalopod molluscs, e.g. squid and octopus. It is perhaps not surprising therefore that these animals have extremely well-developed nervous systems, albeit based on the general molluscan plan of central ganglia and peripheral plexuses. However, cephalopods contain many more ganglia than other molluscs, most of which have fused to form a complex brain mass around the oesophagus. Ganglia are also found peripherally in these animals as swellings on the nerves which emanate from their central nervous systems.

## 2.7   Vertebrates

The vertebrate central nervous system develops in the embryo from a flat plate of tissue which invaginates to form a neural tube. Early in development the front end of the neural tube enlarges to take the form of three primary vesicles, the presumptive forebrain (prosencephalon), midbrain (mesencephalon) and hindbrain (rhombencephalon). The rest of the neural tube persists to the adult stage as the spinal cord.

The spinal cord, which is dorsal in position and is the least specialized part of the vertebrate central nervous system, usually consists of a rod of material, invested by a thick membranous wall, with a thin canal running down the centre, but in agnathous fish, e.g. *Myxine*, the spinal cord is flattened and ribbon-like. Segmentally arranged nerves, called spinal nerves, arise from the lateral walls of the spinal cord. It seems likely

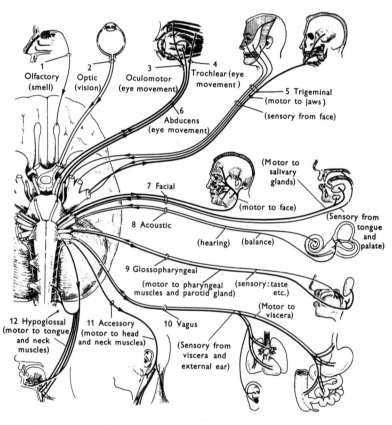

**Fig. 2–4**  Twelve pairs of cranial nerves arise from the ventral surface of the human brain to supply the head, neck and viscera. Other vertebrates also have twelve pairs of cranial nerves with very similar functions and identical names. (From MCNAUGHT & CALLANDER, 1970, after F. H. NETTER. The Ciba Collection of Medical Illustrations.)

that, primitively, there were two pairs of spinal nerves per segment, one dorsal nerve and one ventral nerve on either side, but in all living vertebrates the dorsal and ventral nerves have fused, although their roots are still present. Segmental nerves also arise from the brain, although cephalization has obscured their segmental origins (Fig. 2–4). These are called cranial nerves and most of them are homologous with the spinal nerves, except that fusion of dorsal and ventral nerves has not occurred in the brain as it has in the spinal cord. Some of the brain nerves, for example, the olfactory nerve which innervates the snout, although they are called cranial nerves, are not segmental nerves.

The presence of a ganglion on the dorsal root of the spinal nerve is an important characteristic of the vertebrate central nervous system. This is called the dorsal root ganglion and contains the somata of afferent neurons. The afferent neuron is monopolar, its single axon process branching as it leaves the dorsal root ganglion, one branch passing into the spinal cord, the other branch passing down the dorsal root to the spinal nerve and thence to the sensory structure of which it is part (Fig. 2–5).

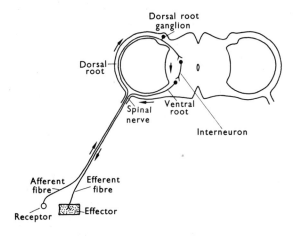

**Fig. 2–5**   Most reflex arcs in man involve at least three sets of neurons, sensory neurons, motor neurons and one or more sets of interneurons.

The somata of motor neurons and interneurons are located centrally in the spinal cord, where they form a dense core surrounded by a peripheral rind of axons, i.e. the converse of the arrangement seen in the invertebrate nerve cord. In transverse section the spinal cord appears to be divided into a central H-shaped zone, which is grey in appearance and which contains somata and unmyelinated neuron processes, surrounded by a white zone containing mainly axons with their myelin sheaths. The former is called grey (gray) matter, the latter white matter. Glial cells lie in the spaces between the neurons. The somata of motor neurons lie in the ventral horns (corona) of the grey matter and send axons out of the cord to the effectors via the ventral roots. Processes from sensory or afferent neurons may make direct synaptic contact with motor neurons to form a simple reflex arc (Fig. 2–6). More usually, the sensory and motor nerve cells are connected by one or more interneurons (Fig. 2–5) the somata of which are mainly in the

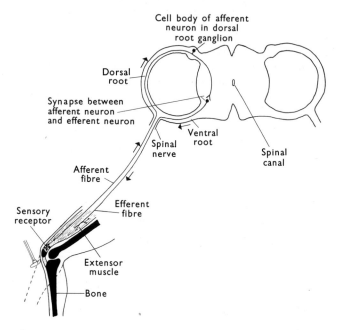

**Fig. 2–6** The human knee jerk reflex involves only two sets of neurons and is initiated by tapping the patellar tendon which stretches the extensor muscle in the thigh. This in turn stretches the muscle spindles (not shown) in this muscle and messages from these receptors, together with messages from sensory receptors in the tendons, are transmitted to the spinal cord by afferent fibres. The afferent fibres synapse with motor neurons in the spinal cord and information transferred from the sensory neurons to the motor neurons causes the extensor muscle to contract. (After MCNAUGHT & CALLANDER, 1970.)

dorsal horns (equivalent to posterior horns in man) of the grey matter. Some of the interneurons are intrasegmental. Others are intersegmental and send axons up and down the cord to connect up the motor and sensory systems of the different spinal segments. A third group of interneurons connect the spinal neurons with neurons in the brain.

From the central nervous system (brain and spinal cord) the cranial nerves and spinal nerves, which can be said to constitute the major part of the peripheral nervous system, pass out to muscles, glands, sense organs etc. The spinal nerves are mixed nerves and contain many thousands of efferent and afferent axons. In mammals there are thirty-one pairs of spinal nerves but in some amphibians (e.g. the frog), where the spinal cord is short, there are only ten pairs of spinal nerves.

## 2.8  The vertebrate brain

It must be emphasized that the vertebrate brain is just an elaboration of the front end of the embryonic neural tube and, as such, it has many features in common with the spinal cord. White and grey matter are present, and the central canal found in the spinal cord extends into the brain where in parts it has expanded to form large spaces or ventricles. In fish, the wall of the brain is like that of the spinal cord, i.e. with inner grey and outer white zones, but in parts of the brains of higher vertebrates, for example in the cerebral cortex of man, some of the somata of the grey matter have migrated outwards to form a third layer on top of the white, axon zone.

### 2.8.1  FOREBRAIN

The anterior of the forebrain is called the telencephalon, the posterior part the diencephalon (Fig. 2–7). In all vertebrates except fish a pair of cerebral hemispheres (cerebrum) arises from the dorsal surface of the forebrain, the paired corpora striata forming the floor of these structures, and during development the telencephalon becomes drawn out to form paired olfactory lobes. In mammals the cerebral hemispheres become very large and the development of structures as the dominant region of the brain reaches its zenith in man. The surface area of the cerebral hemisphere is greatly increased in mammals by the formation of superficial furrows or sulci (Fig. 2–7). The outer surface of the cerebral hemispheres consists of a thin (3 mm) layer of grey matter known as the cerebral cortex (Plate 1) and this becomes the area in mammals to which most sensory information is sent (Fig. 6–9), and which dominates and co-ordinates voluntary activities and also some involuntary activities. The cerebral cortex transmits motor commands to other parts of the brain and to the spinal cord via special pathways, the pyramidal tracts (Fig. 6–10).

The cavity in the hind end of the forebrain is expanded to form the third ventricle and it communicates with the cavities in the cerebral hemispheres, i.e. the lateral ventricles, by the Foramen of Munro. In some vertebrates part of the roof of the third ventricle is vascular and is called the choroid plexus, while the lateral walls of this ventricle form the thalamus on either side. The floor of the third ventricle forms the hypothalamus, which is an important autonomic centre for the regulation of smooth muscle, cardiac muscle and certain glands.

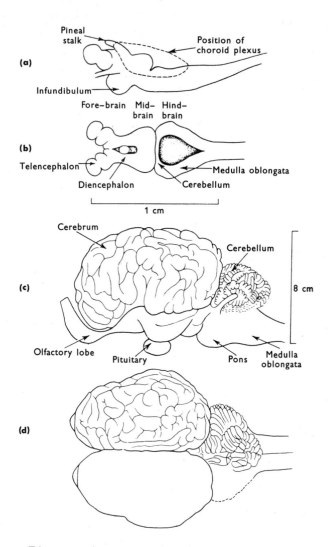

**Fig. 2–7**   Diagrammatic representation of the lamprey brain in (a) lateral view and (b) dorsal view illustrating the gross structure of a relatively simple vertebrate brain. Lateral view (c) and dorsal view (d) of the brain of the horse. Note extensive development of the cerebrum and cerebellum. (From WOOD, 1968.)

## 2.8.2   MIDBRAIN

Whereas the vertebrate forebrain is primitively concerned with smell, the midbrain is primitively an optic centre. In lower vertebrates the optic nerves from the eyes pass straight through the diencephalon after decussating (crossing-over) at the optic chiasma. The optic fibres end in a primary visual centre in the roof (optic tectum) of the midbrain, which is swollen to produce two or four (corpora quadrigemina) optic lobes. Since fish do not have cerebral hemispheres (Fig. 2–7) it has been suggested that the optic tectum in these animals is analogous to the cerebral cortex of higher vertebrates. The forebrain of amphibians shows some of the dominance which is so characteristic of the mammalian forebrain, but even here the midbrain is still an important integrative centre and it is not until we reach the reptiles that a conspicuous shift in dominance occurs, with the appearance of a cerebral cortex.

## 2.8.3   HINDBRAIN

The anterior roof of the hindbrain is enlarged to form a structure varying greatly in size in different animals and known as the cerebellum (Fig. 2–7). The cerebellum is quite large in mammals and most fish, where it consists of two cerebellar hemispheres, but is usually small in amphibians and reptiles. In mammals the cerebellum is principally concerned with the proprioceptive co-ordination of muscular activity. The floor of the mammalian hindbrain is thickened to form the pons anteriorly and the medulla oblongata posteriorly, the latter merging with the spinal cord. The mammalian midbrain, pons and medulla oblongata are often referred to collectively as the brain stem. A striking feature of the medulla oblongata of fish and amphibians is the presence of two giant neurons, called Mauthner neurons, with large axons which extend the entire length of the spinal cord. Giant neurons are frequently also found in invertebrates (in a transverse section of the earthworm ventral nerve cord one medial and two lateral giant axons can be seen) and, like Mauthner neurons, they are usually employed during 'escape' modes of behaviour, but they are not found in reptiles, birds and mammals.

In the lower vertebrates connections between the different parts of the brain are rather restricted, but during evolution there has been an elaboration and multiplication of nerve tracts linking the various parts of the brain and this has resulted in qualitative and quantitative changes in the activity of some of these parts. In addition to these tracts, a network of neurons and nerve tracts, known compositely as the reticular formation, has developed. This is found in the central area of the brain, particularly in the pons, medulla oblongata and diencephalon. It is the main motor outlet from the cerebral cortex and it also receives much sensory information. As such it appears to be of importance in controlling consciousness, lesions in the various parts of the reticulum resulting in permanent sleep or coma.

## 2.9   Autonomic nervous systems

Most vertebrates possess an autonomic nervous system consisting of a series of ganglia united by commisural nerves and giving off nerves and nerve branches to the viscera. In mammals the autonomic system innervates smooth muscle, cardiac muscle and glands. The activities of these effectors are regulated, but not triggered by, two sets of efferent neurons, sympathetic and parasympathetic. These efferent autonomic pathways each contain two peripheral neurons for the conduction of motor information

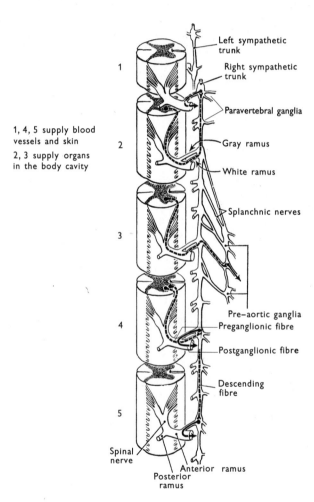

Fig. 2–8   Diagrammatic representation of part of the human sympathetic nervous system from the right side. (From BASMAJIAN, 1964.)

from the central nervous system to the effectors, one preganglionic, the other postganglionic. A ganglionic chain containing sympathetic neurons is found on either side of the vertebral column in which the spinal cord is located, and there are sympathetic fibres running in the spinal nerves and cranial nerves (Fig. 2–8). In man, cells lying in the lateral horn of the thoracic segments and the first three lumbar segments of the spinal cord send efferent, preganglionic fibres to the sympathetic ganglia, and these synapse with postganglionic neurons, the somata of which reside in the sympathetic ganglia. From the sympathetic ganglia postganglionic fibres run to the effectors. The preganglionic fibres are myelinated and the postganglionic fibres are non-myelinated. The sympathetic and parasympathetic nervous systems also send axons out along the cranial nerves.

PARASYMPATHETIC NERVOUS SYSTEM IN MAN

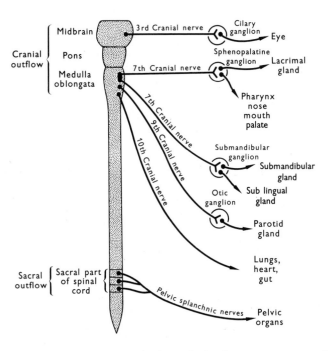

**Fig. 2–9** Diagrammatic representation of the human parasympathetic nervous system. The somata of the primary or preganglionic neurons of the parasympathetic system are found in two widely separate regions of the central nervous system. Some are in the brain stem and others are in the sacral portion of the spinal cord. For this reason the parasympathetic nervous system is generally referred to as the cranio-sacral outflow. (From BASMAJIAN, 1964.)

Perhaps the best known cranial autonomic outflow is the tenth cranial nerve or vagus nerve, which innervates the lungs, heart and gut and contains both sympathetic and parasympathetic fibres (Figs. 2–4, 2–9). The parasympathetic outflow from the brain stem consists of preganglionic fibres which, with the exception of those in the vagus nerve, synapse with postganglionic neurons in parasympathetic ganglia sometimes located on the effectors. Processes from the postganglionic neurons innervate the effectors. The preganglionic parasympathetic fibres in the vagus and pelvic splanchnic nerves pass directly to effectors and synapse in the walls of these end organs with postganglionic neurons, which in turn innervate the effectors.

The arthropod visceral or stomatogastric nervous system resembles the vertebrate autonomic system in some respects. It innervates heart and gut muscle, the reproductive system, many glands and the endocrine system. The nervous supply to the arthropod alimentary canal consists of up to four paired nerves originating from the circumoesophageal connectives. It contains sensory and motor fibres and there are a number of associated peripheral ganglia. In some arthropods the rhythmic activity of the heart is controlled by its intrinsic nervous system, consisting of a group of interacting ganglion cells lying on the surface of the heart. These generate rhythmic bursts of activity which initiate contraction of the heart muscle. This activity of the ganglion cells is influenced by information, travelling along segmental nerves from the central nervous system, which may augment or inhibit the output from the ganglionic system. Hormones, for stimulating and regulating a variety of physiological and developmental processes, are produced by neurosecretory neurons as well as by endocrine organs, neuronal and endocrine functions being closely allied in arthropods.

Modern electrophysiology, of which the physiology of nervous systems or neurophysiology is part, is based on the concept that nerve cells are capable of generating, storing and releasing electrical energy and that these properties reside, in the main, in the surface membrane which separates the neuron from its extracellular environment. The excitable properties of neurons are usually described in terms which are more familiar to the physicist and physical chemist than to the biologist and it is necessary to have a basic knowledge of electrochemistry in order to fully appreciate the ways in which nerve cells operate.

## 3.1 Introductory electrochemistry

The solids or liquids, through which electrical energy or electrical current will readily pass can be divided into two types, metallic conductors, such as the metal wires that convey electricity from domestic fuse boxes to electric light sockets, and electrolytic conductors, such as solutions of salts (electrolytes). The movement of electricity through a metallic conductor occurs without transfer of matter in the conductor, the current being transferred by negatively charged particles called electrons. In electrolytic conductors electric current is carried by much larger particles, called ions, which are of atomic or molecular size and are either positively charged (cations) or negatively charged (anions). For example, the salt, sodium chloride, forms two ions; its sodium atoms acquire positive charges by losing electrons while its chloride atoms gain electrons and thereby acquire negative charges. When sodium chloride is dissolved in water the sodium and chloride ions lead more or less independent lives, although they are attracted to each other, to some extent, by virtue of the opposite charges that they carry. Some water molecules will tend to accumulate around the sodium and chloride ions to form shells (hydrated layers) of water molecules.

If two wires (electrodes) of similar composition are dipped into a beaker containing a solution of sodium chloride in water, electric current will not spontaneously flow through the electrolyte between the electrodes when the circuit is completed by connecting the wires outside the beaker. It is undoubtedly true that the sodium and chloride ions are in continuous thermal motion in the electrolyte at this time, but their movements are highly disorganized (Fig. 3–1a). However, if the electrodes are connected to the terminals of a battery, the electrode connected to the positive terminal becomes covered with positive charges while the other electrode becomes covered with negative charges. The positive electrode is said to have a positive potential and is called an anode; the negative electrode is said to

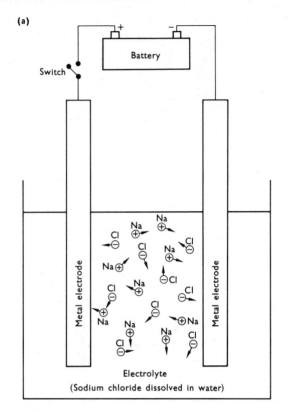

**Fig. 3–1** (a) An aqueous solution of sodium chloride contains sodium and chloride ions undergoing random chaotic motion. When two similar metal electrodes are placed in the electrolyte this state of affairs remains unchanged. However, when, as in (b), the electrodes are connected to a battery by a closing switch, one electrode becomes positively charged and attracts the negatively charged chloride ions, while the other electrode becomes negatively charged and attracts the positively charged sodium ions. The movements of these ions through the electrolyte towards the electrodes constitutes a flow of electric current.

have a negative potential and is called a cathode. In other words, the electrodes become extensions of the battery terminals, the potential difference that develops between them depending mainly on the electromotive force (voltage) of the battery. The sodium ions in the electrolyte are attracted to the cathodal electrode, while the chloride ions by virtue of their negative charges are attracted to the anodal electrode. This bi-directional movement of charged particles through the electrolyte constitutes a flow of electricity, the cations representing positive current, the anions representing negative

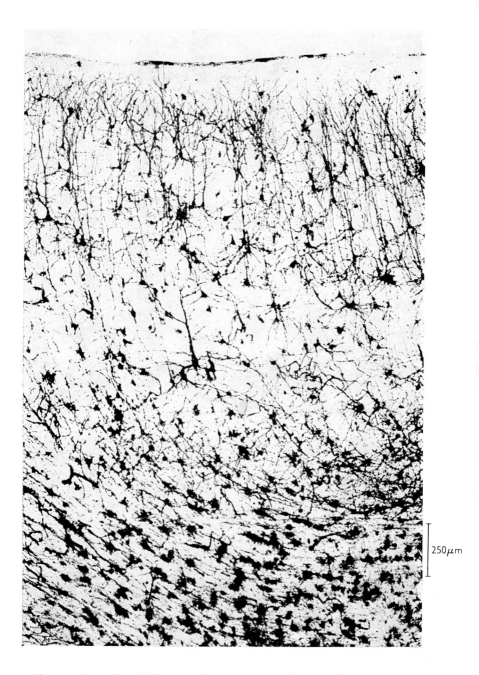

250μm

**Plate 1**  A section of the sensori-motor cortex of the cat illustrating the complex neuron structure and arrangement. Since only about 1·5 % of the neurons in this section are stained by the mercuric chloride-dichromate stain that was employed, the complexity of this part of the cortex is obviously quite staggering. (From SHOLL, 1956.)

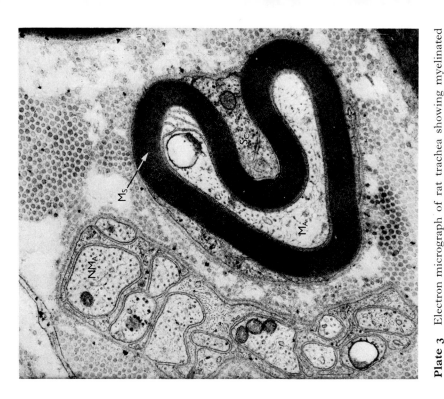

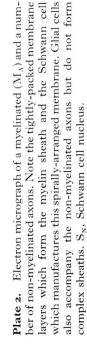

**Plate 3** Electron micrograph of rat trachea showing myelinated nerve fibres in the adventitia. M$_A$, myelinated axon; M$_S$, myelin sheath; NM$_A$, non-myelinated axon; S$_C$, Schwann cell.

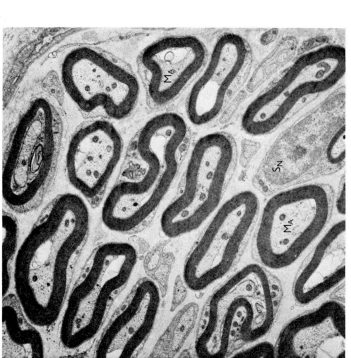

**Plate 2.** Electron micrograph of a myelinated (M$_A$) and a number of non-myelinated axons. Note the tightly-packed membrane layers which form the myelin sheath and the Schwann cell which manufactures this spirally-arranged membrane. Glial cells also accompany the non-myelinated axons but do not form complex sheaths. S$_N$, Schwann cell nucleus.

(Plates 2 and 3 were kindly supplied by Dr. K. J. Ballard, Depart-

**(b)**

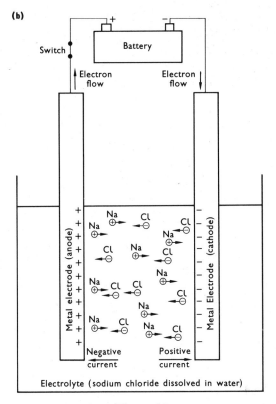

(Fig. 3–1b)

current (Fig. 3–1b). The magnitude of this current will depend on a variety of factors including the potential difference between the two electrodes, the size of the electrodes and the number of ions in solution (this depends mainly on the concentration of the electrolyte). Current will also flow through the metal wires to and from the battery but in the form of electrons rather than ions. At the interfaces between the electrodes and the electrolyte rather complex chemical reactions can occur, but discussion of these is outside the scope of this book. It is sufficient for our purposes to assume that when a sodium ion arrives at the cathodal electrode it recovers its lost electron, by taking one of the free electrons present on the surface of the electrode, and becomes a sodium atom once again. The electron lost by the cathode is immediately replaced by the battery, the anode of which can be considered as a store of electrons. At the anodal electrode the chloride ions relinquish their extra electrons to the electrode and become chloride atoms, the relinquished electrons neutralizing some of the positive charges on the electrode surface. Under certain conditions this process will continue until the battery's store of available energy has been depleted.

It might seem reasonable to assume that when current flows through an aqueous salt solution the positive and negative ions will move at the same rate, albeit in different directions. Unfortunately it is not quite as simple as this because ions differ in size and mass and in the number of water molecules that they attract and have, therefore, to drag along with them. For example, sodium ions are smaller than chloride ions yet, because they have a bigger shell of water molecules, they move more slowly through the electrolyte. The sodium ion is said to have a lower mobility than the chloride ion across the neuron membrane.

If a dilute solution of sodium chloride is carefully poured into a beaker containing a concentrated solution of this salt, so that the dilute solution forms a layer on top of the concentrated solution, there will be a tendency for sodium and chloride ions to pass into the more dilute component and for water to pass into the concentrated component. These movements constitute a process called diffusion. Since sodium ions have a lower mobility than chloride ions they will tend to lag behind, causing a slight separation of the charges carried by the anions and cations. As a result, at the boundary or interface between the dilute and concentrated solutions, a layer of positive charges will appear on one side of the boundary and a layer of negative charges on the other side. This separation of charges, or Electrical Double Layer, results in a potential difference which, because it arises from free diffusion, is called a diffusion potential. This potential difference cannot be easily measured under the above conditions but it may be considerable since sodium and chloride ions carry relatively enormous charges. However, if the dilute and concentrated salt solutions are separated by a well-defined boundary, which allows them to mix only very slowly, it is then possible to obtain a relatively accurate measure of the diffusion potential.

If a $10^{-1}$ molar solution of sodium chloride is placed in a porous pot and the pot is then surrounded by a solution of $10^{-2}$ molar sodium chloride (Fig. 3–2) there will be a net efflux of sodium and chloride ions through the wall of the pot from the concentrated to the dilute solution and a net influx of water. However, since sodium ions move more slowly than chloride ions an Electrical Double Layer will be set up in the wall of the pot, resulting initially in a potential difference of about 12 mV, with the inside of the pot positive with respect to the outside. As the two solutions slowly equilibrate this potential difference will fall towards zero. Even when equilibration has been achieved and the concentrations of sodium and chloride ions are the same in both compartments, these ions will still move in and out of the pot, but in the absence of a concentration gradient for sodium chloride the numbers of ions entering and leaving will be the same and there will be no net separation of charge and therefore no potential difference across the wall of the pot. Potential differences can arise, therefore, by the spontaneous mixing of aqueous salt solutions of different concentrations,

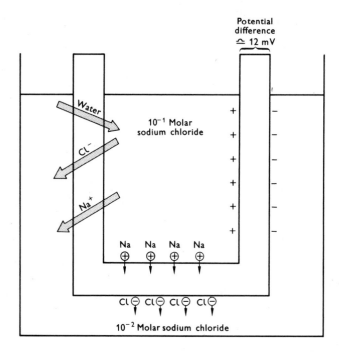

**Fig. 3–2** A $10^{-1}$ molar solution of sodium chloride has been placed in a porous pot surrounded by a $10^{-2}$ molar solution of this salt. The wall of the pot is equally permeable to sodium ions and to chloride ions and there is, therefore, as illustrated on the left hand side of the diagram, a net efflux of these ions from the porous pot. However, since chloride ions have a greater mobility than sodium ions, they tend to move faster and this results in a slight, but significant, separation of anions from their co-ions. This is illustrated at the bottom of the diagram. This separation of charge initially produces a potential difference across the wall of the pot, as indicated on the right hand side of the diagram.

containing ions with different mobilities. The magnitude of the potential difference that will appear under these conditions will be determined by how much these concentrations and mobilities differ and can be expressed by the equation:

$$E = \frac{u - v}{u + v} \cdot \frac{RT}{nF} \ln \frac{C_1}{C_2} \qquad (1)$$

Where $E$ = potential difference
$\quad\quad\ R$ = the gas constant
$\quad\quad\ T$ = absolute temperature

$F =$ the Faraday constant

$n =$ ion valency

$C_1$ and $C_2 =$ concentrations of the salt solutions outside and inside of the porous pot

u and v $=$ mobilities of cations and anions respectively

(At $18°$ C the mobility of sodium ion $= 4 \cdot 5$ cm$^2$ V$^{-1}$ s$^{-1} \times 10^{-4}$ and the mobility of chloride ion $= 6 \cdot 8$ cm$^2$ V$^{-1}$ s$^{-1} \times 10^{-4}$.)

It is apparent from equation (1) that the magnitude of the potential difference could be altered by changing the mobility of either one or both of the ions in the electrolyte so that the charge separation across the wall of the pot is either greater or less than before. One way to affect the rate of migration of an ion is to physically impede its progress by placing a membrane in its path. We shall consider the special case where the mobility of one of a pair of ion species is reduced to zero by a membrane which is impermeable to that ion species. If the pores of a porous pot are filled with a precipitate of copper ferrocyanide a potential difference of about 58mV can be obtained across the wall of the pot by filling the pot with $10^{-1}$ molar potassium sulphate and placing it in a $10^{-2}$ molar solution of this salt (Fig. 3–3).

The copper ferrocyanide membrane prevents sulphate ions from either leaving or entering the pot (the sulphate ions are said to be impermeant) but provides no impediment to the movement of potassium ions. The potassium ions, therefore diffuse down their concentration gradient from inside to outside of the pot through the membrane, but in doing so they become separated from sulphate co-ions. As a result a potential difference appears which eventually opposes any further separation of charge. The potassium sulphate as a whole is indiffusible owing to the electrostatic attraction between its ions. However, dilution of the contents of the pot and concentration of the surrounding solution will still occur through osmotic movement of water across the membrane, but this will be opposed by the development of a hydrostatic pressure, as the volume of fluid in the pot increases. Eventually an equilibrium, called a Donnan equilibrium, will be attained and the potential difference across the membrane will then be a true equilibrium potential. Since this potential difference is due to the diffusion of potassium alone it is a special kind of potassium diffusion potential, i.e. a potassium equilibrium potential.

We can conclude therefore that when two salt solutions containing similar ion species are separated by a membrane, the potential difference between the two solutions will be determined by the differences in the concentrations of the ions on the two sides of the membrane, by the relative rates of migration of these ions through the membranes and by the charges that they carry, i.e. their valencies. In order to differentiate between the rate of migration of ions in a solution and their rate of migration through a membrane the term permeability is assigned to the latter, the term mobility being restricted to the former. For monovalent ions:

$$E = \frac{RT}{F} \ln \frac{C_o + \alpha A_i}{C_i + \alpha A_o} \qquad (2)$$

Where $C_o$ and $C_i$ = external and internal concentrations of cations
$A_o$ and $A_i$ = external and internal concentrations of anions

$$\alpha = \frac{\text{anion permeability}}{\text{cation permeability}}$$

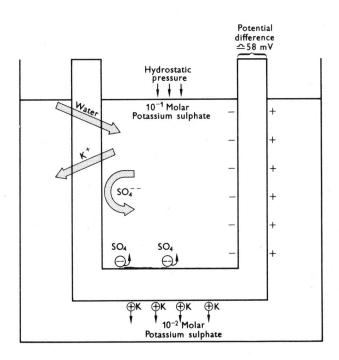

**Fig. 3-3** A $10^{-1}$ molar solution of potassium sulphate is separated from a $10^{-2}$ molar solution of this salt by a copper ferrocyanide membrane contained in the wall of a porous pot. This membrane is permeable to potassium ions but not to sulphate ions (see left hand side of diagram). The potassium ions tend to diffuse down their concentration gradient, across the membrane, to the outside of the porous pot, but are prevented from actually doing so by the impermeance of their sulphate co-ions. Nevertheless a slight separation of potassium ions from sulphate ions does occur (see bottom of diagram) and this sets up a potential difference across the membrane as illustrated on the right hand side of the diagram.

## 3.2  Electrochemistry of neurons

From the point of view of its electrical properties the neuron is best described in terms of three major components, the extracellular environment, the intracellular environment and the membrane. Since nerve cells do not contain metallic conductors we must assume that the electrical currents that they generate are carried by ions in aqueous solution.

### 3.2.1.  THE MEMBRANE

One of the basic concepts on which modern ideas of electrobiology are based is that there is a thin surface barrier or membrane which controls the diffusion of substances in and out of a cell. It has been suggested, on the basis of chemical analyses and experimental studies, that the neuronal membrane, like membranes of many other cells, contains phospholipids and proteins arranged in a bimolecular lipid (fat) leaflet within a protein framework (Fig. 3–4). Unfortunately it has not been possible to test this suggestion in any meaningful way, since the neuron membrane is so thin that it cannot be seen with the light microscope and conclusively identified. With some fixation techniques a thin structure bordering the neuron can be demonstrated with the electron microscope. This is about 7·5 nm thick and consists of two outer parallel electron dense zones and an inner, less electron dense zone, and has been termed a 'unit' membrane. Possibly the outer zones represent the charged (polar) hydrophilic heads of phospholipid molecules, with associated protein molecules, which form the so-called bimolecular leaflet referred to earlier, the inner zone possibly representing the uncharged (non-polar) hydrophobic parts of the phospholipid molecules. In order to gain further insight into the structural and physiological properties of cell membranes attempts are being made to simulate them 'in vitro'. Artificial membranes made from pure lipid can be

**Fig. 3–4** (a) Hypothetical structure of the neuron membrane showing a bimolecular lipid leaflet with protein-lined pores of different sizes. A possible explanation for the 'unit membrane' seen by microscopists is illustrated. The distribution of ions on the two sides of the membrane is represented schematically. It is assumed that they move randomly in all directions and that an ion can pass through the membrane pores provided that it either fits exactly (i.e. either its hydrated or crystalline diameter is identical to the pore diameter) or that it is slightly smaller than the pore and has a charge which is opposite to that of the surface material lining the pore. Other possible lipid configurations with aqueous pores are illustrated in (b) and (c) where lipid molecules are arranged in either circular (b) or spherical (c) micelles. These configurations could produce a membrane with a discontinuous hydrocarbon phase, which could account for the granular membranes seen by some electronmicroscopists. Membranes not only surround the cell cytoplasm, but they also make up a large part of the internal structure of the cell and may account for 40–90 % of the total cell mass. They are also the site of much enzymic activity. The ions are represented by their relative hydrated diameters.

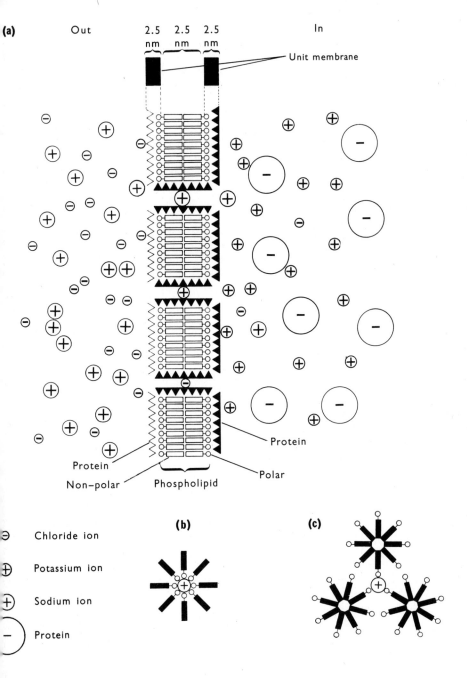

manufactured quite easily. Lipid membranes are practically impermeable to inorganic ions but when they absorb proteins their resistance to these ions is greatly reduced. Possibly the protein molecules penetrate the lipid and form aqueous channels in the membrane through which the ions can pass. Quite recently artificial lipid membranes have been 'seeded' with proteins from natural membranes and, as a result, it has been possible to transfer some of the specific permeability properties of a natural membrane to an artificial membrane.

If we assume that movement of water and ions across the membrane of the nerve cell occurs through hydrophilic channels, possibly lined with protein, bearing positive and negative charges, then the nature of the charge on the walls of these channels could determine which class of ions are able to pass through them, i.e. cations would enter negatively charged channels, anions would enter positively charged channels. In this way membranes with different permeability properties could be produced. Of course the diameter of a channel would also play a role in determining which ions pass along it. One important point to remember is that the membrane of the nerve cell is not a semi-permeable membrane like, for example, cellophane, which merely holds back most solutes while allowing water to pass through. The neuron membrane is a selectively permeable membrane which favours the passage of some species of ions more than others.

3.2.2   INTRACELLULAR AND EXTRACELLULAR ENVIRONMENTS

The cytoplasm of a neuron is composed of 80–90% water. The rest consists mainly of proteins, free amino acids and inorganic salts. The watery environment outside the neuron is of somewhat similar composition apart from its low protein and low free amino acid content. Nevertheless there are important differences in the distribution of specific inorganic ions in the extracellular and intracellular phases. In the extracellular phase chloride is the major anion and its concentration here is about ten times higher than in the cytoplasm of the neuron. This unequal distribution of chloride is possibly due to the presence of large, impermeant organic anions (e.g. isethionate) in the cytoplasm which results in a Donnan equilibrium with chloride as the permeant ion of the Donnan system. Although there is evidence that chloride ions are distributed passively between the extracellular and intracellular environments according to a Donnan equilibrium, there is no evidence that the distributions of sodium and potassium ions arise in this way, yet sodium is about ten times more concentrated outside than inside the cell whereas the intracellular concentration of potassium is approximately 20–50 times higher than the extracellular concentration of this ion. It is more likely that asymmetries in the cation distribution are due to the activity of 'pumps' in the surface membrane of the nerve cell, which transport sodium out of the cell and potassium into the cell. These are energy requiring processes believed to be dependent upon the availability of adenosine triphosphate (ATP). There is good evidence that in some neurons the sodium and potassium pumps are coupled, so that for every sodium ion transported out of the cell a potassium ion is transported inwards. In view of the supposed metabolic dependence of these ion transport processes it is probably not surprising that they can be effectively blocked by metabolic inhibitors such as dinitrophenol (Fig. 3–5). Active transport of ions across neuronal membranes can by itself produce an electrical potential difference across these membranes. For example, in the absence of an opposing potassium pump, an outward sodium pump would produce a 'positive-outside' potential difference, since a pump effectively separates the ions that it transports from their co-ions. An uncoupled pump is said to be an electrogenic pump, whereas the 1:1 coupled sodium-potassium pump referred to earlier is electrically neutral.

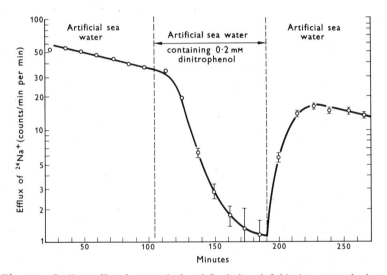

**Fig. 3–5**  Sodium efflux from an isolated *Sepia* (cuttlefish) giant axon during treatment with dinitrophenol (DNP), an inhibitor of oxidative metabolism (production of ATP inhibited with resultant failure of sodium pump). Abscissa: time after end of electrical stimulation of axon in sea water containing radioactive sodium ($^{24}$Na). Ordinate (logarithmic scale) rate at which $^{24}$Na leaves axon. Vertical lines are $\pm 2 \times$ standard error of mean. Experiment was conducted at 18°C. The axon was first loaded with labelled sodium by stimulating it in a solution containing $^{24}$Na. It was then superperfused with saline containing unlabelled sodium and samples of the fluid which flowed past the axon were collected at intervals and counted. The samples contained some labelled sodium which was pumped out of the axon interior across the axon membrane, but the amount of $^{24}$Na appearing in the extracellular fluid decreased with time, due to depletion of the intracellular sodium. Note that the rate of sodium efflux is reversibly inhibited by DNP. (From HODGKIN & KEYNES, 1955.)

In summary then, concentration gradients for sodium, potassium and chloride ions exist across the membrane which borders the nerve cell. We shall find that the nerve cell can generate a variety of different membrane potentials by varying the relative permeabilities of these ions and that in doing so electric currents are caused to flow across the membrane and through the extracellular and intracellular environments of the neuron.

## 3.3   Resting membrane potential

The resting membrane of the nerve cell is highly permeable to potassium ions, usually somewhat less permeable to chloride ions and much less permeable to sodium ions (Fig. 3–6). In view of this and in view of the concentration gradients which exist for these ions, it follows that there will be a potential difference across the membrane and that the magnitude of this potential difference will be mainly determined by the magnitude of the potassium concentration gradient. In other words the potential difference will approach the potassium equilibrium potential, i.e.:

$$E = \frac{RT}{F}\ln\frac{[K]_o}{[K]_i} \qquad (3)$$

where $[K]_o$ and $[K]_i$ = extracellular and intracellular potassium concentrations. A more accurate assessment of the resting potential can be obtained by using equation (2) and taking into account the concentrations and relative permeabilities of sodium, chloride and potassium. Potential differences of 50–90 mV can be recorded from many different neurons when these cells are at rest, i.e. not generating electrical signals. These potential differences are called resting membrane potentials.

## 3.4   Generation of electrical signals

The resting membrane potential is produced by differences in concentrations of potassium ions (and possibly also chloride ions and, to a much lesser extent, sodium ions) in the extracellular and intracellular environment of this cell and by the relative permeabilities of these ions (Fig. 3–6). The inorganic ion concentration gradients across the neuron membrane represent stores of potential energy. We shall find that the neuron utilizes these energy stores to generate electrical signals. Under certain conditions changes in either the ionic concentration gradients or the permeabilities of sodium, potassium and chloride will result in changes in the membrane potential. Although the neuron cannot easily change the ionic content of its two environments, especially at the rate and to the extent that would be necessary to influence the membrane potential, it can change the ionic permeability properties of its membrane. For example we

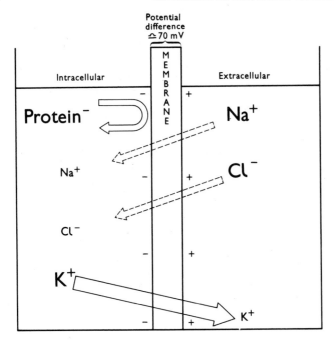

**Fig. 3–6** Schematic representation of the electrochemistry of a resting neuron. The intracellular environment of the neuron is represented by the contents of the left compartment, the membrane of the neuron by the membrane separating the two compartments and the extracellular environment of the neuron by the contents of the right compartment. The left compartment contains high concentrations of potassium ions and negatively charged protein particles, but low concentrations of sodium and chloride ions, whereas the reverse is true for the right compartment. The membrane is very permeable to potassium ions, less permeable to chloride ions, slightly permeable to sodium ions and impermeable to the organic anions. As a result, the potassium, chloride and sodium ions will tend to move down their concentration gradients and a potential difference will be set up across the membrane. Since potassium is the most permeant ion the diffusion of this ion will contribute most to this *resting* potential. The sodium and potassium pumps which maintain the concentration gradients for these ions are not included in the diagram.

shall find that sequential changes in sodium and potassium permeabilities produce electrical signals called action potentials, and that changes in either sodium, potassium or chloride permeability (or possibly a combination of such changes) lead to the appearance of receptor and generator potentials in sensory systems and to the generation of synaptic potentials at synapses etc.

## 3.5   The ionic basis of the action potential

According to the hypothesis propounded by A. L. Hodgkin and A. F. Huxley in 1939 the action potential arises from a large transitory increase in sodium permeability of the neuron membrane, when the membrane potential is reduced (depolarization) below a critical level (threshold) by current flowing outward across the neuron membrane. For a brief period the sodium permeability far exceeds that of other ions, with the result that, the membrane potential changes from inside negative to inside positive, as sodium ions move down their concentration gradient into the neuron. The increase in sodium permeability, or sodium activation, lasts for about 0·5 msec (Fig. 3·7). The mechanisms responsible for this change in membrane

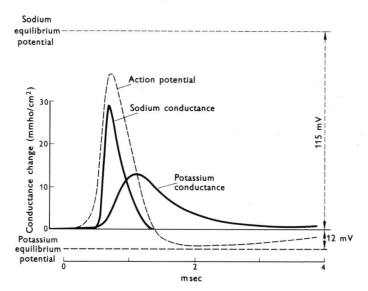

**Fig. 3–7** Calculated changes in sodium conductance and potassium conductance during a theoretical propagated action potential at 18·5°C.
Temperature has a large effect on the rate at which the permeabilities to sodium and potassium change and in this way controls the form of the action potential. (After HODGKIN & HUXLEY, 1952.)

permeability are unknown, but once the change has occurred, another 1 msec must elapse before it can be repeated. This accounts for the observed refractoriness of nerve cells referred to later in this chapter. Shortly after the start of sodium activation a slow increase in potassium permeability occurs. This is called potassium activation and it reaches a maximum when the sodium permeability has almost returned to normal (sodium inactiva-

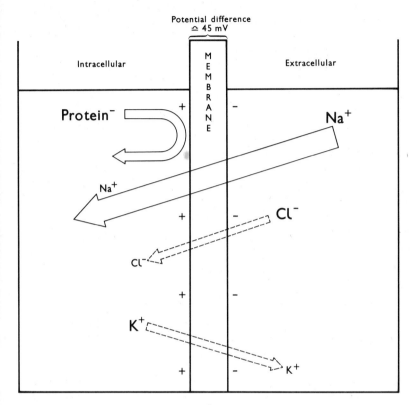

**Fig. 3–8**   Schematic representation of the electrochemistry of an active neuron. For simplicity we shall assume that all parts of the membrane are simultaneously generating an action potential and that the action potential has reached its peak. The sodium permeability greatly exceeds the potassium permeability at this time, and the membrane potential is mainly due to diffusion of sodium down its concentration gradient. Distribution of ions in extracellular and intracellular environment same as for Fig. 3–6.

tion). Potassium activation accounts for the rapid repolarization of the axon membrane which terminates the action potential. At the peak of the action potential, since the sodium permeability at this time is so high, the potential difference across the neuron membrane approaches the sodium equilibrium potential (Fig. 3–8) and in many neurons can be predicted on the basis of the sodium concentrations outside $[Na]_o$ and inside $[Na]_i$ the neuron according to the equation:

$$E = \frac{RT}{F} \ln \frac{[Na]_o}{[Na]_i} \qquad (4)$$

When the action potential has reached its peak, sodium inactivation produces a rapid fall in sodium permeability, and with the continuing rise in potassium permeability, the potential difference across the neuron membrane quickly returns towards the potassium equilibrium potential. If the potassium equilibrium potential does not coincide exactly with the resting potential then, for a short time (a few msec), the membrane potential will be either slightly more negative or less negative than the resting potential. This transient deviation of the membrane potential from its resting value is called an after-potential. Eventually the potential difference across the membrane returns to its resting value, as the potassium permeability falls to its resting value (potassium inactivation).

During the generation of an action potential a small amount of sodium enters the neuron and a small amount of potassium leaves the cell. However, a single action potential never increases the internal sodium concentration by more than about $10^{-6}\%$, and this is quickly removed by the sodium pump. Even when the pump is rendered inoperative by metabolic inhibitors such as dinitrophenol (Fig. 3.5) a neuron can still produce many hundreds of action potentials before the sodium and potassium concentration gradients are significantly affected.

## 3.6   Passive electrical properties of neurons

The neuron membrane is often likened to an electrical circuit comprising many repeating units. Each unit is said to contain a number of batteries, one for each species of ion (Fig. 3–9), the electromotive forces of these batteries being determined by the concentration gradients for the different ions. In the electrical analogue of the neuron membrane each ionic battery is connected between the extracellular and intracellular phases by a variable resistance, which represents the permeability of the membrane to the species of ion concerned. The resistance is variable rather than fixed because we have seen that when the neuron is generating electrical signals, the perme-

Fig. 3–9   Electrical analogue or equivalent circuit of a neuron membrane at rest (a), at the peak of an action potential (b), and during the repolarization phase of an action potential (c). The differences in ion concentrations across the neuron membrane are represented by batteries; the electromotive forces of these batteries are dependent upon the concentration gradients for the specific ions. The permeability of the neuron membrane to specific ions is represented by resistances placed in series with the batteries. Since the permeability properties of the membrane change during activity, the resistances are of the variable type. During the peak of the action potential (b) the sodium permeability is very high and this is denoted by a fall in the sodium resistance. As a result the potential difference across the cell membrane is now mainly determined by the electromotive force of the sodium battery. At rest and during repolarization, the potassium resistance is lowest and the potential difference is determined mainly by the electromotive force of the potassium battery.

abilities of some ions, especially sodium and potassium, change consider-
ably. Since the membrane separates electrical charges it must also behave
as a capacitor. In fact, the capacity of the neuron membrane is about
1 uF/cm² and electrical current flows in and out of this capacitor when the
neuron generates electrical signals. Although electrical analogues of the
neuron membrane must not be taken too seriously, they do provide a
simplified description of the electrical properties of the membrane. Of
course, according to Fig. 3–9, the inside of the neuron is connected to the
outside through resistances and since these are not infinite there is no

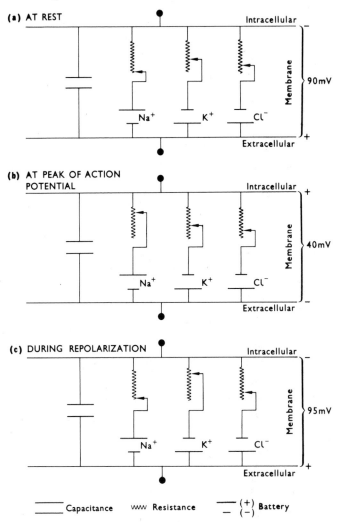

reason why the ionic batteries should not run down. Indeed, the ionic batteries of the neuron membrane are continuously discharging as the permeant ions, sodium and potassium move down their concentration gradients, but they are also being simultaneously recharged by the sodium and potassium pumps which work to maintain the concentration gradients for these ions.

The longitudinal flow of current through the cytoplasm of the neuron is determined by the conductivity of the cytoplasm and the transverse resistance afforded by the neuron membrane. Since the neuron membrane is a rather 'leaky' structure and, therefore, has a relatively low resistance, it follows that the passive longitudinal spread of current is usually very restricted. Indeed, subthreshold currents spread over only short distances, often no more than a few mm, and the potentials (electrotonic potentials) that they set up become distorted and attenuated with distance, because of current loss through the leaky membrane and energy dissipation in the cytoplasm, membrane and extracellular fluid (Fig. 3–10). In an axon the ratio of the transmembrane resistance/axoplasmic resistance decreases more or less exponentially with increasing distances along the axon from a fixed point and, therefore, the preferential pathway for current is normally always across the near membrane. The situation for dendrites and cell bodies is somewhat more complex than this because of their more complicated architecture. Axons are often many cm long and electrical transmission of information over such distances by subthreshold signals would be impossible. Therefore, some other form of signal must be employed. The neuron has solved this problem by regenerating signals at every point along the length of its axon.

---

**Fig. 3–10**   Electrotonic potentials and action potentials recorded from an isolated axon. An intracellular stimulating electrode is used to pass pulses of either inward current (a) or outward current (b) across the axon membrane. The resultant hyperpolarizations (a) or depolarizations (b), recorded by three intracellular recording microelectrodes, are illustrated in records 1–3 in (a) and (b). Traces marked 'stimulus' indicate the polarity and amplitude of the applied current pulses. Note that inward current pulses produce only hyperpolarizing electrotonic potentials which 'spread' more or less instantaneously along the axon in a decremental fashion, so that the potentials at recording electrode No. 1 are smaller than those at recording electrode No. 2, while no potentials are recorded at electrode No. 3. With outward current pulses, depolarizing electrotonic potentials result from pulses of low current intensity and these 'spread' along the axon with decrement. However, when the depolarizations reach the critical threshold, one or more action potentials are initiated and these are recorded by all three recording electrodes, the response height being identical at all three recording sites. This is because all-or-none action potentials are conducted along the axon without decrement. However, they are conducted relatively slowly along the axon and as a result there are measurable delays between arrival of an action potential at the different electrode sites.

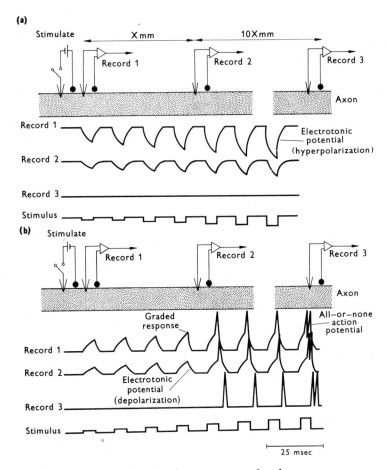

## 3·7   The action potential and nervous conduction

If a pair of non-polarizable electrodes are placed against an axon and a square pulse of current (stimulus) is passed between the electrodes, by transiently making one electrode positive and the other negative, most of the current will flow in the extracellular fluid between the electrodes, if this is a low resistance pathway. However, some of the current will flow across the axon membrane in an inward direction at the positive electrode (anode) and in an outward direction at the negative electrode (cathode). As a result of the outward flow of current at the cathode the membrane capacitance is transiently discharged at this point and the potential difference at this point falls towards zero. At the termination of the stimulus the membrane repolarizes and the membrane capacitance is recharged. Opposite changes occur at the membrane under the anode. Here the inward current increases the potential difference across the axon membrane. This is called hyperpolarization and it is also followed at the termination of the stimulus by return of the membrane potential to its resting value. Although the stimulus pulse may have a fast rise time and decay time, the response of the axon membrane follows a relatively slow (exponential) time course dependent upon the time constant of the membrane (its resistance × its capacitance). If the stimulus strength is low, then these are the only changes which occur and the electrotonic potentials which are set up at the two electrodes 'spread' almost instantaneously along the axon, declining as they do so, due to the leaky properties of the membrane (Fig. 3–10). These electrotonic potentials are set up by 'local circuit action', i.e. longitudinal spread of current (Fig. 3–11).

If the membrane under the cathode is subjected to a depolarization exceeding about 20 mV the permeability properties of the membrane at this site are transiently altered. The magnitude of the current which must flow across the neuron membrane before this change will occur is called the threshold current, while the membrane potential at which it occurs is called the threshold voltage or critical depolarization threshold. As soon as the membrane is depolarized beyond the critical depolarization threshold a regenerative change occurs and, for an instant, the inside of the membrane becomes 35–45 mV more positive than the outside. The membrane potential then quickly returns to its resting value. This sequence of events produces the action potential (spike, impulse) and usually lasts for about 1 msec. The changes in membrane potential which occur during the action potential cannot be controlled by changing the stimulus intensity. Once the critical depolarization threshold is exceeded, an action potential occurs and its height is, under certain conditions, always the same; if the critical depolarization threshold is not reached, then no action potential is initiated. For this reason the action potential is said to be an all-or-none or all-or-nothing response.

After initiating an action potential under the cathode electrode, a second response cannot be initiated at this same site within a period of about 1 ms, no matter how strong one makes the second stimulus. The period during which a second action potential cannot be evoked is called the absolute refractory period and it corresponds to the period of sodium inactivation referred to earlier. It is followed by the relative refractory period, lasting for 5–10 msec, during which the nerve cell recovers its excitability and the critical depolarization threshold is higher than normal. Following the relative refractory period there is often a period of heightened excitability, called the supernormal phase. Refractoriness ensures that the action potential is a discrete signal and that there is no overlapping of events, but it does impose certain limitations on the frequency of occurrence of this type of signal (firing frequency). The maximum frequency which is theoretically possible is somewhat less than 1000/sec, although this is rarely

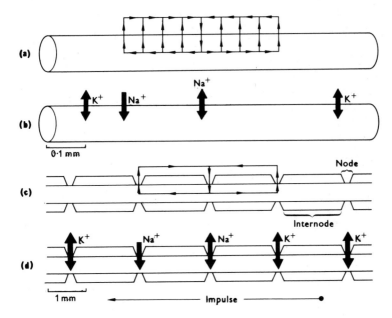

**Fig. 3–11** Nervous conduction in a non-myelinated axon (a and b) and a myelinated axon (c and d). The electrical currents associated with an all-or-none action potential are illustrated in (a) and (c) while the ionic movements are illustrated in (b) and (d). In the non-myelinated axon unidirectional conduction is ensured by transitory refractoriness of previously active regions of the neuron membrane. The insulating sheath, which invests the myelinated axon, restricts the local currents which flow across the neuron membrane mainly to the nodes and, as a result, the action potential is initiated only at these sites. Conduction is, therefore, achieved by a series of jumps, i.e. it is salatory. Once again, refractoriness ensures that conduction of the action potential is unidirectional. The ionic mechanisms underlying the generation of an action potential are the same for both types of axon. The length of the myelinated axon illustrated in (c–d) must be envisaged to be many times greater than that of the non-myelinated axon in (a–b). Arrows indicated net movements of ions; double-headed arrow indicates ion as in electrochemical equilibrium.

achieved, frequencies up to 200/sec being much more usual. An interesting effect of refractoriness is seen when two action potentials are generated, one at one end, the other at the other end of an axon, and propagated towards the centre of the axon. When these responses meet or collide they are both eliminated since the site of the collision is completely surrounded by membrane which is in the refractory state.

With the exception of a few specialized regions most of the neuron membrane is capable of generating action potentials. When such a response is initiated at one end of an axon under a cathodal electrode, the change in potential difference across the membrane at this site causes currents to flow in local circuits from the activated region along the inside of the axon, outward across the membrane, back towards the activated zone in the extracellular fluid and inward across the activated membrane (Fig. 3–11). The outward flow of current across membrane immediately adjacent to the activated site is quite intense and usually sufficient to depolarize this membrane beyond the threshold for initiation of an action potential. This in turn generates local currents which flow in both directions along the axon. The membrane under the cathodal electrode does not produce another action potential in response to this new current flow because it is refractory at this time; only the region in front of the newly activated zone responds in this way. As a result of this, an action potential is conducted along the axon in one direction only. If, however, the cathodal electrode is placed halfway along the length of the axon, then two action potentials will be generated by the local currents set up by the stimulus and these will be conducted in both directions away from the stimulated site. The action potential travels along the nerve at a rate far slower than that of light or sound in a similar medium. The velocity of the action potential depends upon the passive electrical properties of the axon. The longitudinal resistance of the axoplasm is one important determinant and this is influenced by the diameter of the fibre, in the same way that the resistance of a wire is inversely proportional to the square of its diameter. In giant axons ($\approx$ 1 mm diam.), the local circuit currents spread much further longitudinally than in normal size axons because of the relatively low resistance afforded by their axoplasm. Local currents associated with an action potential generated at one site in the giant axon membrane are effective in depolarizing quite distant regions beyond their critical depolarization threshold. In fine non-myelinated axons (0·001– 0·1 mm diam.) the local circuit currents associated with an action potential are restricted by the high resistance of the axoplasm and, therefore, only

---

**Fig. 3–12** Intracellular recordings from a giant axon during extracellular stimulation. The extracellular stimulating electrodes are illustrated on the left of (a–d), the intracellular recording electrode, amplifying and display equipment on the right. In (a), the intracellular electrode is inserted into the axon and the resultant downward deflection of the oscilloscope beam is a measure of the resting potential difference across the axon membrane. In (b), a brief pulse of current is passed between the stimulating electrodes. Some of this flows across the axon membrane and an action potential is initiated under the cathodal electrode. The passage of the current pulse is instantaneously indicated by the appearance of a stimulus artefact on the oscilloscope trace. In (c), the action potential arrives at the recording site and the oscilloscope beam is deflected to register an inside positive potential at the peak of the action potential, In (d), the action potential has passed the recording site and the membrane potential at this site has returned to its resting state. The time taken for the action potential to travel from the cathode to the recording site is indicated by the interval between the stimulus artefact and the beginning of the spike.

regions of membrane immediately adjacent to a spike generating site will be sufficiently depolarized for spike production. As a result, the conduction velocity of the action potential can be as low as 0·5 m/s in fine axons, whereas in giant axons values as high as 100 m/s are not unusual. Giant axons are used for conducting information during escape behaviour when a high conduction velocity is obviously of paramount importance.

In the case of myelinated axons, the velocity of conduction of the action potential is far greater (up to 100 m/s) than their diameter (1–20 μm) would suggest. This is because the myelin sheath is such a good insulator that it effectively limits the current pathway across the axon membrane to the nodes

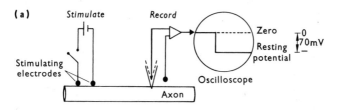

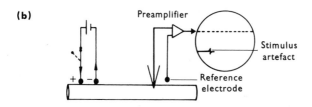

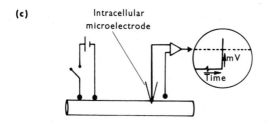

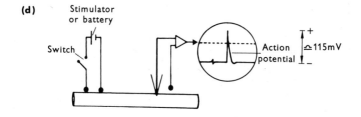

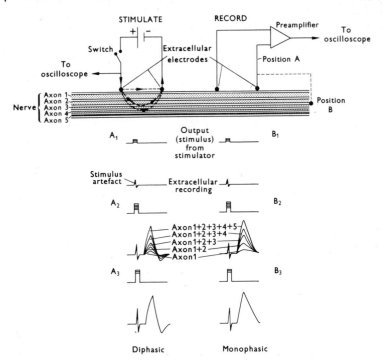

**Fig. 3–13** Schematic representation of extracellular recordings from an isolated frog sciatic nerve during stimulation with extracellular electrodes. The stimuli consisted of square pulses of current of increasing amplitude (top traces, A and B). The sciatic nerve contains many nerve fibres of differing diameter and some of these are represented in the diagram. In (A) the two recordings electrodes were placed close together on the nerve and diphasic action potentials were recorded ($A_2$ and $A_3$). In (B) the distal recording electrode was placed against the cut end of the nerve. As a result monophasic action potentials were recorded ($B_2$ and $B_3$). At the two lowest stimulus intensities no action potentials were elicited (bottom traces $A_1$ and $B_1$). In ($A_2$) and ($B_2$) the stimulus intensity was increased by five discrete steps. A response was recorded each time, the magnitude of the response being related to the stimulus intensity. The action potential increased in height as more and more axons were excited. When all the axons were excited further increases in stimulus intensity did not increase the height of the compound action potential ($A_3$ and $B_3$).

of Ranvier, although there is a slight leak across the myelinated zones or internodes (Fig. 3–12). This means that local circuit currents set up by an action potential occurring at one node will pass along the inside and outside (indeed outside the myelin sheath) of the axon and across the axon membrane of adjacent nodes. It is at these points that the next action potential is generated. In other words the action potential 'jumps' from node to node and that is why this sort of nervous conduction is called 'saltatory'. Unidirectional conduction is assured, as it is in unmyelinated axons, by refractoriness. It is important to remember that all axons can conduct information in both directions, but 'in vivo' conduction is invariably polarized, simply because the neuron is usually stimulated or excited at one end only.

Nerve impulses have now been detected in representatives of the major phyla with the exception of the platyhelminthes and failure here is almost certainly a matter of technical difficulty. Furthermore, neurons usually show the same essential features of all-or-none responsiveness and refractoriness in all animals in which they have been detected.

So far the excitable properties of nerve cells have been discussed in terms of the properties of single axons or neurons. However, the most accessible axons for class experiments are to be found not individually, but collectively in a peripheral nerve such as the sciatic nerve of a frog or a leg nerve of a locust. When a nerve of this type is stimulated by passing current between two extracellular electrodes, the axons that it contains will often appear to have different thresholds for the production of action potentials (Fig. 3–13). Indeed the electrical signal recorded from the sciatic nerve of the frog using extracellular electrodes will be increased in magnitude, often in a stepwise fashion, as more and more axons are excited, by raising the stimulus intensity. The maximum response is called a compound nerve action potential. The apparent differences in threshold of the different axons are due in part to differences in size of axons, which will influence the amount of current which will flow across their membranes, and to the geometry of the system, including the position of the stimulation electrodes. At any one stimulus intensity less current will flow through small axons and axons from the cathodal electrode. These axons will therefore appear to have a higher threshold than large axons and axons close to the cathode. The term threshold, as applied to this system, is somewhat artificial and should not be confused with the current threshold and critical depolarization threshold of neuron membranes referred to earlier. The number of steps which go to make up the compound action potential gives a rough estimate of the number of axons contained in the sciatic nerve. The sciatic nerve of the frog is ideal for demonstrating such fundamental properties of neurons as, for example, refractoriness (Fig. 3–14) and conduction velocity.

## 3.8  Electrophysiological techniques

The techniques used for investigating the electrical properties of a nerve cell are various and quite complex. In order to record the potential difference across a neuron membrane a glass micropipette with a tip diameter of $\simeq 1$ μm is filled with a conducting medium (usually 3M KCl) and is used to

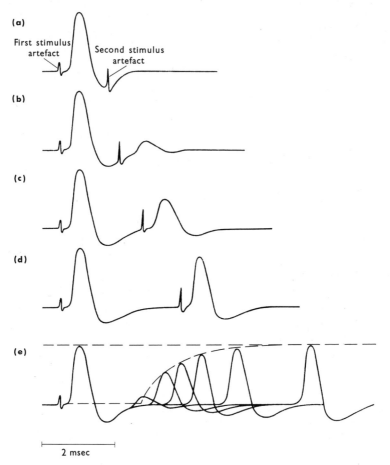

**(a)**

First stimulus artefact

Second stimulus artefact

**(b)**

**(c)**

**(d)**

**(e)**

2 msec

**Fig. 3–14** Demonstration of refractoriness in an isolated whole nerve. In (a) a first stimulus was applied to the nerve through a pair of stimulating electrodes, and a pair of extracellular recording electrodes placed on the nerve recorded a stimulus artefact followed by a large compound diphasic nerve action potential. A second stimulus of identical magnitude and duration was applied during the time of occurrence of this action potential and this second stimulus failed to evoke a response from the nerve. This is because the nerve (or more correctly the axons which it contained) was absolutely refractory at this time (b–c). As the interval between the first and second stimulus was gradually increased a second response appeared which grew in magnitude until it was the same size as the first response. As the interval was increased more and more axons in the nerve became excited a second time. (From KATZ: *Nerve Muscle and Synapse* © 1966 McGraw-Hill Inc. Used by permission.)

penetrate the cell membrane. The microelectrode is connected, by a silver electrode coated with silver chloride, to one input of a DC preamplifier which has a high input impedance. The other input of the amplifier is connected via a second silver/silver chloride electrode either directly to the saline surrounding the nerve cell or via a 'bridge' containing 2% agar in saline. This is the reference electrode and it is often held at earth potential. The output from the preamplifier is connected to the input of the vertical amplifier of an oscilloscope. The potential difference across the neuron membrane is calculated by first determining the potential difference between the two electrodes, when both the reference electrode and the microelectrode are in the saline, and then determining the potential difference after inserting the tip of the microelectrode into the cell. The difference between the two readings is a measure of the potential difference across the neuron membrane. The recording electrode may also be used as an extracellular probe for sampling the currents which flow across the neuron membrane during, for example, an action potential or a synaptic potential. Other microelectrodes can be used either to pass current across the neuron membrane, so that some of the passive and active electrical properties of the cell may be determined, or to inject ions into the neuron in order to investigate its ionic properties. Microelectrodes filled with drugs can be used to test the chemosensitivity of neuron membrane. The drugs are ejected either by pressure or, in ionic form, by electric current. Drug-ejection electrodes are of great value in pinpointing the location of chemically-sensitive sites, e.g. synapses, on the outer surface of the neuron membrane.

The cathode ray oscilloscope is an essential part of an electrophysiologist's equipment. It consists of a cathode which ejects a stream of electrons: a control grid which determines the strength of the electron current and as a result controls the brightness of the oscilloscope trace: a main anode which accelerates the electrons: a focusing anode which forms a sharp electron beam: a pair of horizontal deflection plates, connected to a horizontal amplifier, which drive the electron beam across the face of a fluorescent screen and produce the time axis of a graphical display: a pair of vertical deflection plates which are connected to the vertical amplifier(s). and which give the voltage axis. A metallized screen discharges the electron beam after it has produced a bright spot by collision with the fluorescent screen on the front of the tube. The function of the oscilloscope is therefore to first amplify the signals recorded from the neuron and then to plot these voltage changes or currents against time.

# Synaptic Transmission

When an action potential reaches the axon terminals of a neuron it has, so to speak, reached the end of the line unless the electrical currents which accompany it are capable of generating an action potential in either a second neuron or in an effector cell. This electrical method of intercellular communication does indeed occur at electrical synapses, but at chemical synapses the action potential in a presynaptic cell triggers the release of a chemical from the axon terminals and it is this substance which mediates transmission of information between the presynaptic and postsynaptic elements.

## 4.1 Chemical synapses

### 4.1.1 THE PRESYNAPTIC ELEMENT AND EXCITATION-SECRETION COUPLING

In some neurons, the axon terminals are invaded by the all-or-none action potential which arrives at the terminals after travelling down the axon from the soma. In other neurons, the action potential stops just before it reaches the axon terminals, the axon terminal membrane being informed of its arrival by the depolarization it experiences due to the local currents set up by the pre-terminal spike. In both types of neuron, the net result is a transitory release of a chemical from the axon terminals into the synaptic cleft. The process which couples excitation or depolarization of presynaptic membrane to release of transmitter from the axon terminal is called excitation-secretion coupling. The nature of this process is still very much a mystery although it is known that calcium ions play an important role. If chemical synaptic transmission is to occur at all, then obviously transmitter must be readily available for release into the synaptic cleft when the presynaptic membrane is depolarized. It has been frequently, if somewhat tentatively, suggested that transmitter is stored in the presynaptic vesicles (Fig. 4–1). This is a very convenient idea since it could explain why the transmitter is released in packets or quanta containing a large number of molecules rather than as individual molecules.

In the absence of a nerve impulse small amounts of transmitter are released spontaneously from the nerve terminals. It has been proposed that this occurs because the synaptic vesicles are continuously in motion and that they release their contents into the synaptic cleft when they contact an active site or transmitter release site on the presynaptic membrane. Electron micrographs showing synaptic vesicles in close juxtaposition to the presynaptic membrane, and even apparently opening into the synaptic cleft, have been obtained quite frequently, but it must be emphasized that so far there is no definitive evidence for the release of

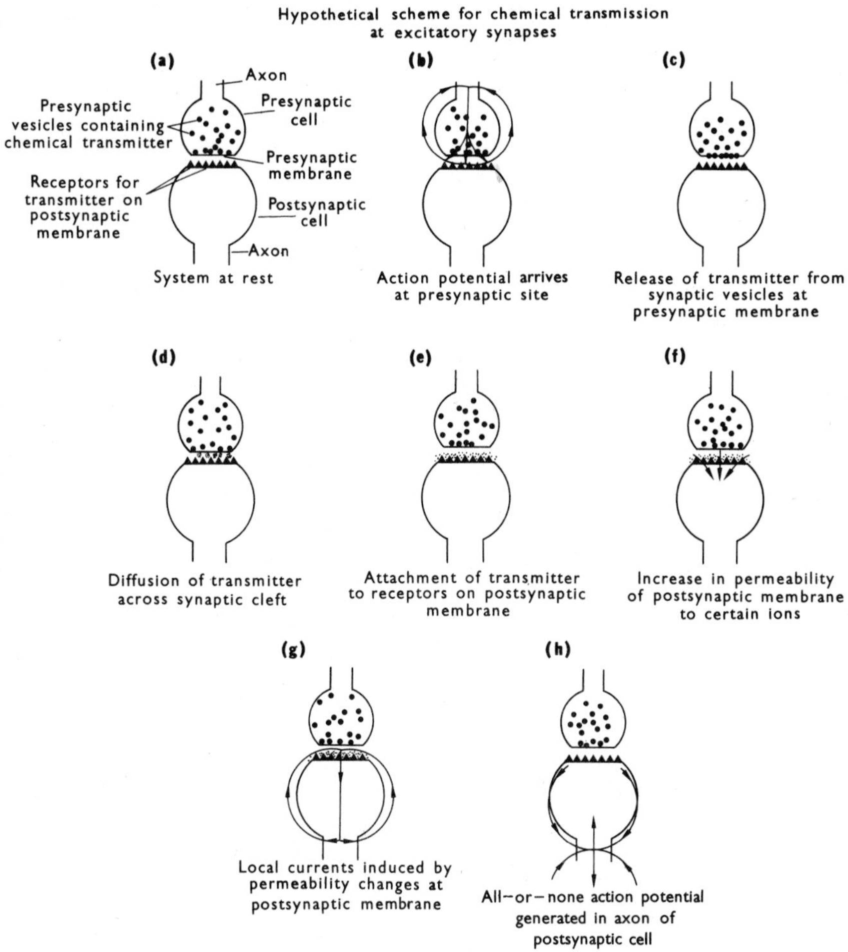

Fig. 4-1 Diagrammatic representation of a hypothetical scheme for chemical transmission at an excitatory synapse between two neurons. (a) Resting synapse. (b) An action potential arrives at the presynaptic terminal and current flows across the presynaptic membrane. As a result the probability of synaptic vesicles releasing their contents into the synaptic cleft is dramatically increased (see text). The transmitter diffuses across the synaptic cleft (d) and reacts with receptors on the postsynaptic membrane (e). This alters the permeability of the postsynaptic membrane and the resultant inward current across this membrane causes current to flow outwards across the spike generating membrane of the postsynaptic cell (g). If an action potential is generated, this in turn sets up local currents which flow back into the soma of the postsynaptic cell and also into the axon of this cell (h).

transmitter from these structures and that there are a number of equally plausible hypotheses for the release of transmitter which exclude the synaptic vesicles altogether. According to the vesicle hypothesis, depolarization of the presynaptic membrane dramatically increases the number of release sites, so that the probability of a vesicle coming into contact with such a site is greatly increased and, as a result, a large number of packets of transmitter are released more or less simultaneously from the axon terminals (Fig. 4–1). Normally depolarization of the terminals lasts for only a limited period (about 2 msec) and the enhanced release of transmitter can be considered to follow a similar time course, so that in effect each action potential releases a 'pulse' of transmitter. In the absence of extracellular calcium depolarization of the nerve terminals by the action potential fails to release any extra transmitter, although the spontaneous release of small quantities of transmitter is not abolished. It seems likely, therefore, that calcium is essential for the production of the supplementary release sites which are postulated to appear when the presynaptic membrane is depolarized.

Many different chemicals, including catecholamines, indolalkyamines and amino acids are used by neurons as transmitters. Acetylcholine is undoubtedly the best known transmitter. This substance is released by motor neurons that innervate vertebrate skeletal muscle, by vertebrate parasympathetic neurons, and possibly by some invertebrate central neurons and motor neurons. Possibly transmitters are manufactured in the axon terminals, although there is some evidence that they are manufactured in the soma and transported down the axon to the terminals, either via the neurotubules or prepacked in vesicles. The terminals of some neurons that release acetylcholine (cholinergic neurons) are equipped metabolically to produce this transmitter by acetylation of choline (Fig. 4–2a), while the terminals of some arthropod inhibitory motor neurons contain enzymes which catalyse the production of $\gamma$-aminobutyrate, the inhibitory transmitter released by these nerve cells (Fig. 4–2b). The continuous replenishment of transmitter lost from axon terminals is greatly assisted by active uptake of either the transmitter itself or its degradation products from the synaptic cleft after transmission has been effected.

### 4.1.2 THE POSTSYNAPTIC ELEMENT

The transmitter secreted from the axon terminals diffuses across the synaptic cleft towards the postsynaptic membrane (Fig. 4–1). The time taken for the transmitter to be released from the terminals and, more especially, to diffuse across the synaptic cleft is thought to account for the delay between arrival of the electrical signal at the terminals of the presynaptic cell and the appearance of a change in the potential difference across the postsynaptic membrane. This delay, which is about 0·7 msec at synapses on frog skeletal muscle fibres, is called the synaptic delay. When the transmitter reaches the postsynaptic membrane it apparently combines with membranous structures called receptors. These are envisaged as

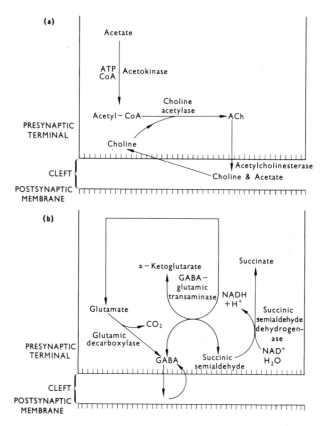

**Fig. 4-2** (a) Scheme for the synthesis and release of acetylcholine (ACh) from the terminals of a cholinergic neuron. (From HUBBARD, LLINÁS & QUASTEL, 1969.)
(b) Scheme for the synthesis and release of γ-aminobutyrate from endings of a crustacean peripheral inhibitory neuron. (From KRAVITZ, MOLINOFF & HALL, 1965.)

chemically defined areas of large molecules which combine with the transmitter by virtue of their chemically complementary nature. The chemical identity of the receptor at cholinergic synapses is currently under intensive investigation and preliminary results suggest that it is a protein containing four sub-units with a total molecular weight of about 80 000. By ejecting minute quantities of transmitter on to very limited areas of the postsynaptic element, it has been demonstrated that the receptors are usually restricted to the postsynaptic membrane and do not extend over the entire membrane of the postsynaptic cell. However, when a muscle fibre or neuron is deprived of its nervous innervation, there is a tendency for the receptors to proliferate over the entire surface of the denervated structure.

The sequence of events which follows or accompanies the reaction of a transmitter molecule with a receptor molecule depends upon the type of synapse, i.e. whether it is excitatory or inhibitory, on the ionic environments of the postsynaptic cell and on the electrical properties of the postsynaptic membrane and non-synaptic membrane of the postsynaptic cell. At a cholinergic synapse on a frog skeletal muscle fibre, acetylcholine reacts with receptor molecules on the postsynaptic membrane and alters the properties of this membrane so that it becomes highly permeable to sodium and potassium ions, but not to chloride ions. The potential difference across the postsynaptic membrane now assumes a new 'equilibrium' value, i.e. intermediate between the sodium equilibrium potential ($\simeq +45$ mV) and the potassium equilibrium potential ($\simeq -90$ mV). This change is accompanied by a flow of inward current across the postsynaptic membrane, the current circuit being completed by an outward flow of current across the adjacent non-synaptic membrane of the muscle fibre (Fig. 4–1g).

In most frog skeletal muscle fibres, the non-synaptic membrane, but not the postsynaptic membrane, is capable of generating all-or-none action potentials when depolarized by outward currents in excess of the threshold current. The postsynaptic membrane can therefore be viewed as a very restricted area of electrically-inexcitable membrane surrounded by a vast area of electrically-excitable or spike generating membrane. Normally the synaptic current is so intense that it always results in depolarization of the immediately adjacent non-synaptic membrane well beyond its threshold for spike production and hence an action potential in the motor neuron is always followed by an action potential in the muscle fibre. The muscle action potential then propagates along the rest of the membrane of the muscle fibre, away from the synaptic site. In this system it is essential that the synaptic potential is followed by an action potential, if the entire contractile system contained within the muscle fibre is to be informed of the arrival of the nerve impulse. This is because the muscle fibres are often many mm in length and each fibre usually makes only one synaptic contact with the motor neuron which innervates it (Fig. 4.3). Since the synaptic currents are restricted to a small area around the synapse it follows that all-or-none action potentials propagating without decrement are required to carry messages to distant regions of a muscle fibre. Other skeletal muscle fibres in the frog and all arthropod skeletal muscle fibres make many synapses with the motor neurons that control them, the synapses being distributed along the entire length of these fibres. This type of innervation is described as multiterminal or distributed. Most muscle fibres with a multiterminal innervation do not need to generate all-or-none action potentials, since all of the surface membrane of these fibres will be affected directly by the synaptic currents generated at the many synaptic sites.

The reaction between acetylcholine and the receptors on the post-

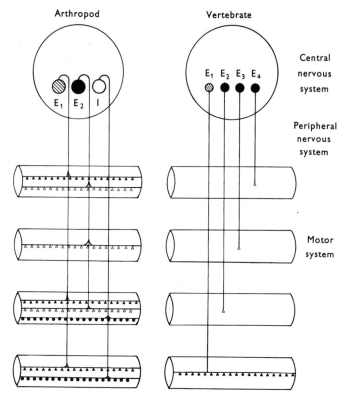

**Fig. 4-3** Diagrammatic representation of the innervation of arthropod and vertebrate (frog) skeletal muscles. Although arthropod muscles may contain many hundreds of muscle fibres they are usually controlled by no more than five motor neurons. Some arthropod muscle fibres are innervated by just one motor neuron, others by more than one motor neuron (polyneuronal innervation). Arthropod motor neurons are of two main types, excitatory (E) and inhibitory (I) and it is the interplay between these neurons that provides for the very fine control of arthropod muscles. The excitatory motor neurons can be roughly subdivided into those that evoke small contractions ($E_1$) and those that evoke big contractions ($E_2$). Most vertebrate skeletal muscles are innervated by many tens of motor neurons, some of which are represented by ($E_2$–$E_4$) which are always excitatory in function. Multiterminal innervation of vertebrate muscle fibres is rare except in some special cases such as frog tonic fibres, which are controlled by 'slow' motor neurons ($E_1$).

synaptic membrane of a frog cholinergic nerve-muscle synapse can be blocked by curare. This substance competes with acetylcholine for the receptors on the postsynaptic membrane, although it does not alter the permeability of this membrane when it combines with the cholinergic receptors. By controlling the amount of curare reaching the synaptic sites, it is possible to produce different degrees of synaptic blockade. When a cholinergic synapse is only partly blocked by curare, the acetylcholine released from the motor nerve terminals by a nerve impulse produces a smaller than normal synaptic potential. The synaptic current associated with this event may not be sufficient to depolarize the non-synaptic membrane beyond the threshold for spike production. The sub-threshold synaptic event appears as a brief depolarization followed by a quasi-exponential repolarization and is called the excitatory postsynaptic potential (EPSP), end-plate potential or junction potential. This response is not all-or-nothing; it does not propagate without decrement and it cannot therefore be recorded at distances of more than a few mm away from the synapse.

The spontaneous release of transmitter from the terminals of frog motor neurons results in the occurrence of sub-threshold EPSP's, rarely exceeding a few mV in amplitude, called miniature potentials. The essential evidence for the quantal nature of the EPSP is in the fact that this response can be fractionated into units, identical in all respects to miniature EPSP's, by raising the magnesium content or lowering the calcium content of the extracellular environment of the synapse. Miniature potentials have been recorded from a variety of vertebrate and invertebrate synapses, where they usually occur randomly in time, although this is not true in every case. Perhaps the temporal distribution of the miniature potentials is related to the spatial distribution of the synaptic vesicles. This would certainly provide attractive support for the vesicle hypothesis.

It now appears likely that the basic essentials of the transmission process at vertebrate cholinergic nerve-muscle synapses are shared by all other excitatory chemical synapses, central and peripheral. The transmitter may well be different and the ions which carry the synaptic current may also differ, but the same quantal process appears to occur. At inhibitory synapses, where transmission is also quantal, reaction between transmitter and postsynaptic receptors usually causes an outward flow of current across the postsynaptic membrane, and a brief hyperpolarization of this membrane and the adjacent non-synaptic membrane. However, at some peripheral inhibitory synapses on arthropod muscle fibres, transmission is accompanied by either no change in potential or even a small depolarization of the postsynaptic membrane. At all inhibitory synapses, the transmitter increases the permeability of the postsynaptic membrane to either potassium and/or chloride ions. The effect of this permeability change on the potential difference across the postsynaptic membrane will depend upon the relationship between the resting potential of the postsynaptic cell, the equilibrium potentials for potassium and/or chloride, which are of course determined by the intracellular and extracellular concentrations of these ions, and on the relative permeabilities of potassium and chloride during the action of the transmitter. At central synapses the net result of inhibitory transmission is that the potential difference across the postsynaptic membrane and adjacent non-synaptic membrane

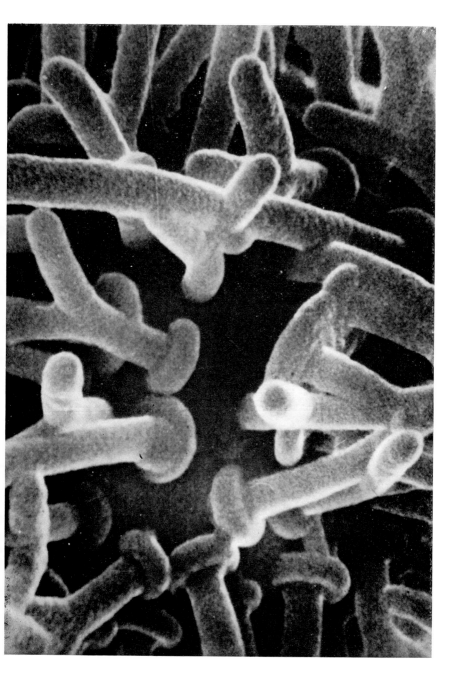

**Plate 4** Nerve terminals forming synapses on somata in an abdominal ganglion of a marine snail. This is a photograph taken with a scanning electron microscope which gives an apparent three-dimensional view of the structure observed. (From *United Press International*, 1970.)

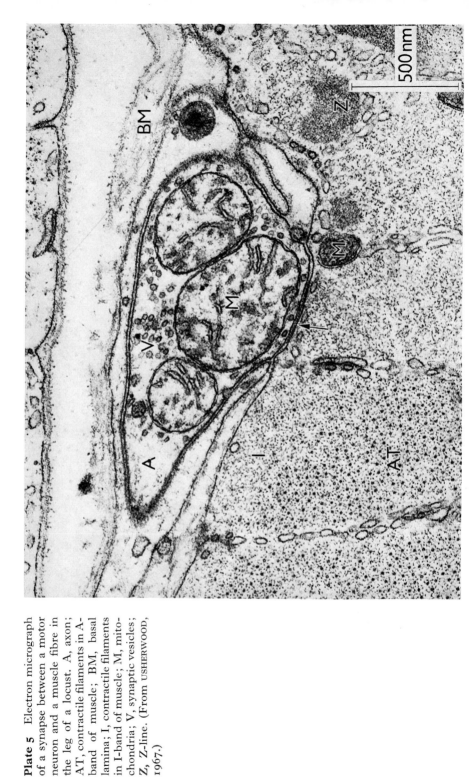

**Plate 5** Electron micrograph of a synapse between a motor neuron and a muscle fibre in the leg of a locust. A, axon; AT, contractile filaments in A-band of muscle; BM, basal lamina; I, contractile filaments in I-band of muscle; M, mitochondria; V, synaptic vesicles; Z, Z-line. (From USHERWOOD, 1967.)

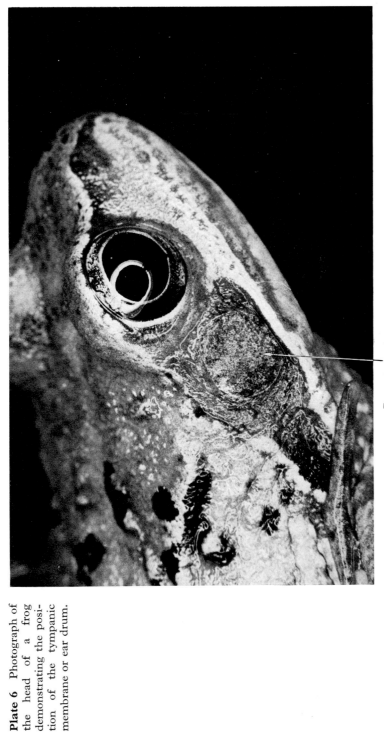

**Plate 6** Photograph of the head of a frog demonstrating the position of the tympanic membrane or ear drum.

Tympanic membrane

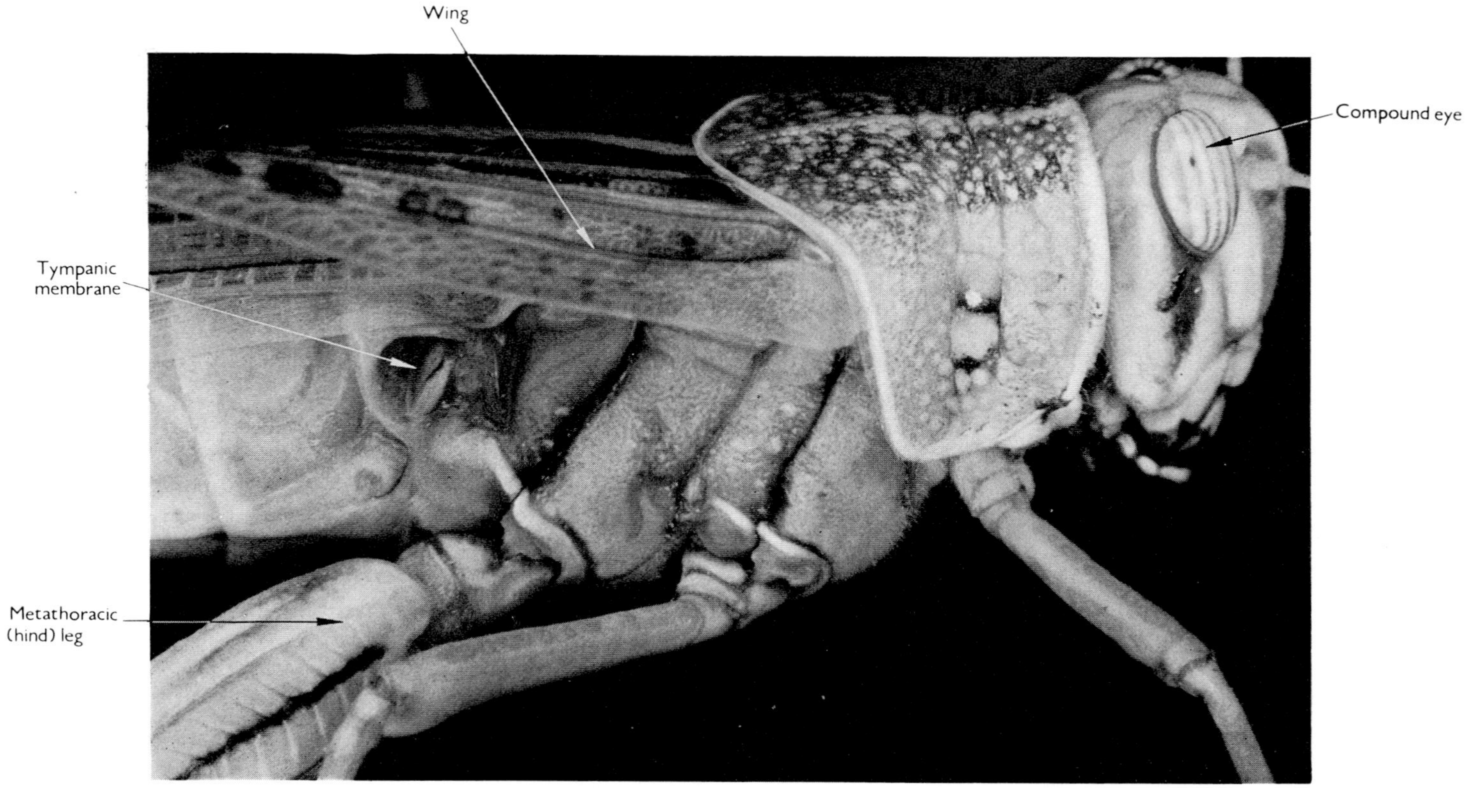

**Plate 7** Photograph of a locust (*Schistocerca gregaria*) illustrating the tympanum on the first abdominal segment and the compound eye on the side of the head.

Compound eye

Wing

Tympanic membrane

Metathoracic (hind) leg

is firmly held, for a brief period, at a level well below the threshold for spike formation, since the equilibrium potentials for potassium and chloride are usually close to the resting potential and this greatly influences the generation of action potentials by the postsynaptic cell. Since arthropod skeletal muscle fibres do not generate all-or-none action potentials, inhibition is expressed as an attentuation of ongoing excitatory activity (depolarization) in the muscle fibres, by the increased conductance of the muscle fibre membrane which accompanies inhibitory synaptic transmission.

Synaptic transmission does not always result in an increase in the permeability of the postsynaptic membrane. At some central synapses in molluscs the transmitter influences the metabolic activity of the postsynaptic membrane by blocking the activity of an electrogenic sodium pump. This results in depolarization of the postsynaptic membrane and excitation of the postsynaptic cell through flow of outward current across the adjacent non-synaptic membrane.

We are left then with the problem of what happens to the transmitter once it has acted upon the postsynaptic membrane. At some synapses it apparently diffuses away and since this could be a relatively slow process, the time course of the transmitter-receptor interaction could be quite prolonged, and a long-lasting synaptic potential could be produced. At other synapses the transmitter is reabsorbed as such by the presynaptic element. This might be either a very fast process or a slow process. In the first case the synaptic potential would be of short duration; in the second case it could be prolonged. At the frog nerve-striated muscle synapse, the acetylcholine released from the terminals of the motor neurons first reacts with the postsynaptic receptors and is then degraded by the enzyme cholinesterase, to choline and acetate. This enzyme is present in the synaptic cleft, usually on the postsynaptic membrane. The choline that is produced is then reabsorbed by the axon terminals. Removal of the transmitter from the synaptic cleft is obviously of great importance since it ensures that the pulses of information conducted along the axon of the presynaptic element can be transferred intelligibly to the postsynaptic element. However, at many synapses simple diffusion of transmitter from the synaptic cleft is probably sufficiently fast to account for efficient removal of transmitter. It seems likely that cholinesterase serves to shorten the time-course of the reaction between acetylcholine and receptor.

There is a wealth of information on the pharmacology of peripheral and central synapses which is beyond the scope of this booklet. Much of this is concerned with the action of drugs on postsynaptic membranes and on the systems which degrade and reabsorb transmitter substances. More recently attention has been turning towards the presynaptic element where it is becoming clear that presynaptic membranes also have many complex pharmacological properties.

## 4.2  Electrical synapses

It has been calculated that depolarization of the postsynaptic membrane of a chemical synapse by the electrical currents associated with the presynaptic action potential rarely exceeds more than 1–2 mV due to leakage of current through the low resistance pathway afforded by the wide synaptic cleft. At electrical synapses or ephapses the resistance of the synaptic cleft is much higher, due to the very close apposition of pre-synaptic and postsynaptic membranes. Therefore a greater proportion of the current associated with the presynaptic action potential crosses the membrane of the postsynaptic cell and the resultant depolarization of the postsynaptic membrane may be sufficient to exceed its depolarization threshold. At electrical synapses the postsynaptic membrane can generate action potentials. Ephapses are usually polarized, so that an action potential in the presynaptic element will induce an action potential in the postsynaptic element, but not vice versa. Inhibitory ephapses also occur, as, for example, on the Mauthner nerve cells of the goldfish. In this case an action potential in the terminals of the presynaptic fibre causes current to flow inwards across the spike generating membrane of the Mauthner neuron. As a result this region is hyperpolarized and the probability that it will generate an action potential is correspondingly reduced. It is interesting to note that ephapses are most frequently associated with escape systems, where undoubtedly the absence of a delay, such as occurs at chemical synapses, is of great importance.

## 4.3  Presynaptic inhibition

At some vertebrate central excitatory synapses and at some synapses on crustacean muscle fibres, the terminals of the presynaptic neuron are innervated by an inhibitory neuron. When this inhibitory neuron is excited, it releases a chemical transmitter, which diffuses across the gap between the terminals of the inhibitory and excitatory presynaptic neurons and interacts with receptors on the terminal of the latter. This transmitter-receptor interaction reduces the resistance of the presynaptic membrane of the presynaptic neuron, so that electrical signals reaching this membrane from the soma of this cell are attenuated and thereby cause less transmitter than normal to be released from the terminals of this neuron. In other words discretely timed inhibitory neuron activity will either partly or completely inhibit the impulse-linked release of transmitter from the excitatory pre-synaptic neuron and thereby partly or completely close the synaptic path-way between this neuron and the postsynaptic element. This phenomenon is called presynaptic inhibition.

## 5.1  General Principles

Since the survival of an animal depends upon its awareness of its external and internal environments, it is perhaps not surprising that most animals are endowed with a remarkably diverse array of sensory structures. Most cells are moderately sensitive to many forms of energy, but sensory receptors are specialized in that they possess enhanced sensitivity to some particular form of energy. However, it is important to carefully distinguish between the specific sensitivity of sensory receptors and the sensations that they create within *our* nervous systems when they are excited. For example, most of our visual sensations arise from the absorption of light energy by sensory receptors in our eyes and it is therefore quite justifiable to term these receptors, photoreceptors. However, the sensation of pain does not result from the reception of pain energy, and it is therefore somewhat misleading to refer to the sensory structures which evoke this sensation as pain receptors.

A sensory receptor is an input element of a nervous system and in its simplest form it consists of a single neuron which has become modified to serve a sensory role. It has one short dendritic process, which is the receptive part of the cell, and an axon process, which either communicates with the rest of the nervous system or communicates directly with effectors (Fig. 5–1). A sensory receptor of this type is called a primary sense cell, because it performs the multiple functions of absorbing some form of environmental energy, transducing it to electrical energy and conducting the resultant electrical information away from the receptive site. The rods and cones of the vertebrate retina are examples of primary sense cells. Sometimes the sensory receptor has a non-nervous origin and in this case it communicates either chemically or electrically with an afferent neuron. A sensory receptor of this type is called a secondary sense cell. Human taste receptors and auditory receptors are examples of this type of sensory receptor. Sensory receptors may occur either as single cells or as small groups of cells. In some cases they are associated with auxiliary structures to form sense organs.

The classification of sensory receptors as either exteroceptors, that collect information impinging upon the integument, or interoceptors, that are located either in or on the internal organs of the body, has been largely superseded by a more convenient classification based on function, in which the sensory receptors are categorized according to the type of stimulus energy to which they are sensitive. For example, there are chemoreceptors for chemical stimuli; mechanoreceptors for movement, pressure, tension,

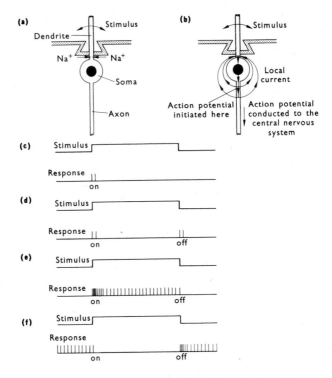

**Fig. 5-1** Ion movements (a), current flow (b) and electrical output (c–f) during excitation of a generalized mechanoreceptor. The sensory receptor is envisaged as a primary sensory neuron. The dendrite process of this cell forms the receptive component of the sensory neuron. Movement of the dendrite, which is ensheathed in an integumental structure, increases its permeability to sodium ions and this leads to a depolarization of the dendritic membrane. As a result, current flows outwards across the membrane of the spike generating region of the axon and action potentials are initiated at this site. The top records in (c–f) indicate the duration of the stimulus while in the bottom records some of the different types of response that can be obtained from mechanoreceptors of this type are illustrated diagrammatically. The ON receptor in (c) generates action potentials only at the beginning of the stimulus; the ON-OFF receptor in (d) only at the beginning and again at the end of the stimulus. These are phasic receptors. The tonic ON-OFF receptor in (e) generates action potentials throughout the entire duration of the stimulus, although there is a gradual decline in spike frequency with time, a phenomenon referred to as adaptation. The output of the ON-OFF receptor in (f) is greatest in the absence of the stimulus, presence of the stimulus being signalled by a decline in spike frequency. It is assumed that in all cases the receptor potential lasts for the duration of the stimulus and that the differences in output result from differences in properties of the spike generating membrane of the sensory neuron (see Fig. 5-2).

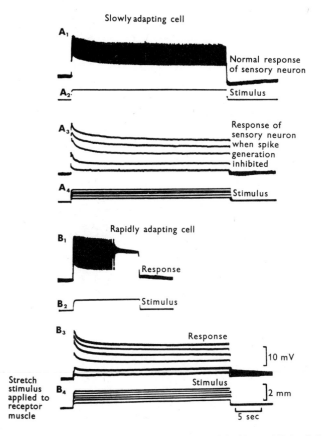

**Fig. 5-2** Spikes (A₁ and B₁) and receptor potentials (A₃ and B₃) of the (A) slow adapting and (B) fast adapting receptor muscles (stretch receptors) of the crayfish in response to stretch stimulation (A₂, A₄ and B₂, B₄). Recordings were obtained by inserting intracellular microelectrodes into the cell bodies of the two sensory neurons. Action potentials are superimposed on the receptor potentials in A₁ and B₁: only the bases of the spikes are illustrated. These recordings were obtained when the receptors were bathed in normal saline. In A₃ and B₃, $2 \times 10^{-7}$ g/cm³ of tetrodotoxin was added to the saline. This drug abolishes spike generation but does not affect the receptor potential. As a result, when the receptor muscles were stretched only receptor potentials were generated. Since the receptor potentials are very similar in both types of neuron, it follows that the differences between the slow adapting cell and the fast adapting cell lie in their spike generating membranes. Scales same for (A) and (B). (From NAKAJIMA & ONODERA, 1969.)

sound and balance; thermoreceptors; electroreceptors for electric fields (in some fishes); and photoreceptors for electromagnetic radiation. The undifferentiated receptors, such as the free nerve endings in mammalian skin which appear to respond to many different types of stimuli, form an additional class.

A sensory receptor transduces any relevant information that it receives from its environment to electrical energy. This transduction process may involve a number of steps, but in all instances the net result is either a transitory depolarization or a hyperpolarization of the receptive membrane due to changes in its permeability to one or more species of inorganic ions. In primary sense cells the change in potential difference across the receptive membrane is called a receptor potential (Fig. 5–2). The amplitude of the receptor potential is proportional to the stimulus intensity and if it is sufficiently large, local circuit action will cause action potentials to be generated in the non-receptive membrane of the sensory neuron (Fig. 5–2) and these will be conducted away from the sensory site along the afferent nerve fibre to other parts of the nervous system. Information about the stimulus is, therefore, pulse-coded in the form of action potentials. Where a sensory neuron receives its information secondhand, so to speak, from a sensory receptor of non-nervous origin, the receptor potential generated by the sensory receptor cell either triggers the release of a chemical transmitter from the sensory receptor, which depolarizes the sensory neuron, or it brings about such a depolarization as a result of direct electrical communication with the sensory neuron. In either event, the depolarization of the sensory neuron is called a generator potential and its amplitude varies with the amplitude of the receptor potential and therefore with the stimulus intensity. If the peak of the generator potential exceeds the depolarization threshold of the sensory neuron, then one or more action potentials are generated. The magnitude of the receptor potential (and therefore the generator potential) is usually a logarithmic function of stimulus intensity, a factor which is of great significance in increasing the range of stimulus intensities to which a sensory receptor can respond. Some sensory neurons generate action potentials throughout the entire duration of even a very prolonged stimulus, whereas others respond only during the initial part of a stimulus. The former are called tonic (static), the latter phasic (dynamic). In both cases the frequency of the action potentials decreases with time, a phenomenon referred to as adaptation (Figs 5–1, 5–2). In some sensory receptors the magnitude of the receptor potential or generator potential declines during a prolonged stimulus and this is reflected, especially in tonic sensory neurons, by a decline in spike frequency. However, in other sensory receptors, such as the stretch receptor of the crayfish, the receptive membrane does not adapt and any decline in spike frequency that does occur results, therefore, from adaptation of the spike generating membrane of the sensory neuron (Fig. 5–2).

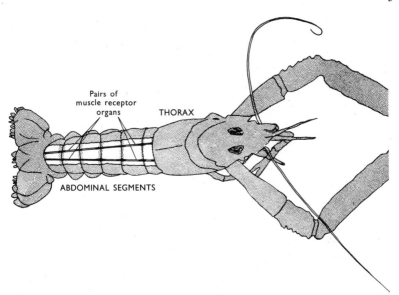

**Fig. 5–3**  Arrangement of some of the muscle receptors in the abdomen of the lobster. A pair of receptors is found in *each* abdominal segment, on either side of the dorsal mid-line, suspended along the longitudinal axis of the segments. The muscle receptors lie on top of the large dorsal extensor muscles of the abdomen and are stretched and excited when the abdomen is flexed.

Some phasic sensory units discharge only a single action potential in response to even a very prolonged stimulus and will remain silent until another stimulus arrives. Sensory receptors of this type are sometimes called on-receptors (Fig. 5–1). Other sensory receptors, called off-receptors, fire an action potential at the end of a stimulus. Yet another group, called on–off receptors, fire at the beginning and again at the end of a stimulus. Less frequently, a sensory neuron may generate action potentials spontaneously and the effect of a stimulus is to increase or decrease (maybe to zero) the frequency of this endogenous activity. Phasic and tonic receptors including on, off, and on–off receptors may occur, side by side, in a single sense organ and, as a result, provide the nervous system with almost the entire information content of a signal.

## 5.2  Mechanoreception

Most mechanoreceptors are designed to respond to low frequency mechanical stimuli. The tactile sensory hairs found all over the bodies of

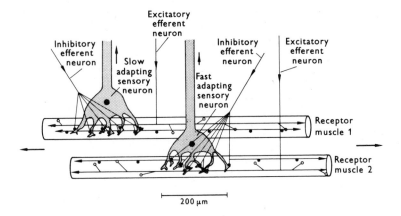

**Fig. 5-4** Diagrammatic representation of a crustacean muscle receptor. Receptor muscle 1 is usually thinner and shorter than receptor muscle 2. Each has a large sensory neuron, the dendrites of which are 'embedded' in a muscle fibre. The dendrites are excited when the muscle receptor is stretched. The dendrites are innervated by endings from an inhibitory neuron which also synapses with the muscle fibre. The muscle fibre is also innervated by one or more excitatory motor neurons.

arthropods and many other animals including mammals, and proprioceptors such as the stretch receptors of crustaceans (Figs. 5-3, 5-4) and the stretch receptors found in vertebrate skeletal muscles (Fig. 5-5) which are of such great importance in posture, locomotion and other co-ordinated movements, are sensory receptors of this type. The pressure sensing elements in human arteries are examples of mechanoreceptors which respond to steady pressure, whereas the auditory receptors of the human ear are examples of mechanoreceptors which respond to high frequency mechanical stimuli.

### 5.2.1 AUDITORY RECEPTORS

The ear of man and other mammals consists of three parts, an external ear, a middle-ear, and an internal (inner) ear (Fig. 5-6). The external ear consists of an auricle or pinna, which is a flap of cartilage covered by skin, and a canal, the external auditory meatus, leading to the middle ear. The pinnae are used, especially in those mammals which can easily move them, to collect sound waves or air vibrations and to direct them into the external auditory meatus. The external ear is separated from the middle ear by a membrane, the tympanic membrane, which is tightly stretched across the end of the external auditory meatus. The outer surface of the tympanic membrane and the surface of the external auditory meatus are lined by skin containing glands which secrete cerumen or ear wax.

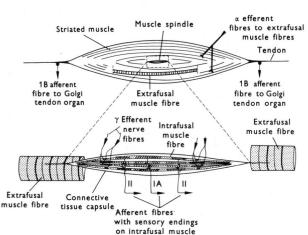

**Fig. 5-5**   A muscle spindle found in vertebrate skeletal muscle. The muscle spindle is contained in a connective tissue capsule and is attached by connective tissue to extrafusal muscle fibres. The spindles contain specialized muscle fibres, called intrafusal fibres, which are supplied with endings from sensory and motor neurons. The sensory endings on mammalian muscle spindles are of two types, primary and secondary. The primary endings form spirals on the centre of an intrafusal fibre. The secondary endings, which lie on either side of the primary endings, may be either spiral in form or they may form sprays of beaded nerve strands. The motor neurons which innervate the intrafusal fibres are called gamma-efferents.

The middle ear is an air-filled cavity containing three bony ossicles which are arranged in series and connect the tympanic membrane to the inner ear. The outermost ossicle or malleus (hammer) is attached to the inner surface of the ear drum and also articulates with the middle ossicle, the incus (anvil). The incus in turn articulates with the innermost ossicle, the stapes (stirrup) which abuts onto an elastic membrane, called the oval window or fenestra ovalis, forming part of the wall of the inner ear. When sound waves impinge upon the tympanic membrane, the ear drum vibrates and the main function of the ossicles is to transmit these vibrations across the middle ear to the inner ear. The ossicles are pivoted in such a way that they are particularly insensitive to vibrations of the head and to bone conducted sound waves. Furthermore the malleus and stapes are attached to the wall of the middle ear by two small muscles, the tensor tympani and the stapedius respectively, and by varying the force developed by these muscles intense vibrations can be attenuated and weak vibrations can be amplified. The middle ear is connected to the naso-pharynx by a tube, the eustachian tube, which functions as a valve to ensure that long-term, and possibly harmful, differences in air pressure on the two sides of the ear

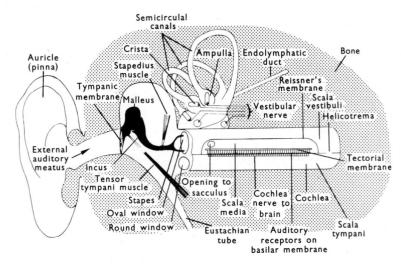

**Fig. 5–6**  Diagrammatic representation of the human ear. The coiling of the
cochlea is not illustrated.

drum do not occur. Transient differences in air pressure which arise when
sound waves impinge upon the tympanic membrane, of course, do not open
and close the eustachian tube.

The inner ear is contained within a series of fluid-filled spaces and
canals, called collectively the bony labyrinth, which are fashioned out of
the periotic bone of the skull. The bony labyrinth contains a fluid called
perilymph and suspended in this fluid is a membranous structure called the
membranous labyrinth. The membranous labyrinth contains a fluid called
endolymph and two types of mechanoreceptors, equilibrium receptors and
auditory receptors. Basically it consists of six interconnected parts, three
semicircular canals, two sac-like structures called the sacculus (saccule)
and utriculus (utricle) and a coiled structure, the cochlea (Fig. 5–7). The
equilibrium receptors are contained within the semicircular canals the
sacculus and the utriculus while the auditory receptors are found in the
cochlea (Fig. 5–8).

The membranous cochlea divides the equally-coiled bony cochlea
longitudinally into three canals. As a result the two outer canals are filled
with perilymph while the inner canal is filled with endolymph. The dorsal
canal or scala vestibuli communicates with the middle ear via the oval
window, while the ventral canal or scala tympani communicates with the
middle ear via a second membrane, called the round window (fenestra
rotunda) which is stretched across a second hole in the bony wall of the
inner ear. At the apex of the cochlea the scala vestibuli and scala tympani
are connected by a duct, the helicotrema (Fig. 5–6). The lateral walls of the

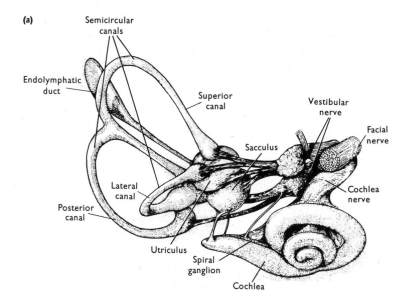

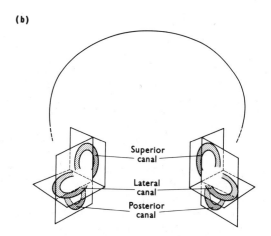

**Fig. 5-7** (a) Human labyrinth and cochlea. (From HARDY, 1935.)
(b) Orientation of semicircular canals viewed through skull from back
towards face. (From WYBURN, PICKFORD & HIRST, 1964.)

membranous cochlea are fused to the sides of the bony cochlea. The dorsal wall of the membranous cochlea forms a thin membrane, called Reissner's membrane (vestibular membrane) while the ventral wall forms a thicker membrane, called the basilar membrane (Fig. 5–8a). The central cochlear duct is called the scala media and it is in this duct that the auditory receptors are located on the inner surface of the basilar membrane, where they form the organ of Corti (Fig. 5–8a). The sensory receptors are arranged in two groups, an inner group and an outer group, which are separated by a perilymphatic duct, the tunnel of Corti. Hair processes from the sensory receptors are embedded in a membrane, called the tectorial membrane, which overlies the organ of Corti.

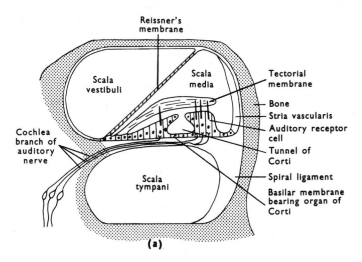

**Fig. 5–8** Sensory receptors of the mammalian ear. (a) Diagram of cross-section of cochlea illustrating structure and position of auditory receptors. (b) Diagram of equilibrium receptors in ampulla of semicircular canal. (c) Diagram of equilibrium receptors on macula of utriculus and sacculus

The manner in which the ear translates sound waves into meaningful auditory messages is not particularly well understood. Vibrations of the ear drum, which are transmitted to the oval window by the ossicles of the middle ear, probably cause disturbances in the perilymph of the scala vestibuli and scala tympani. The membrane of the round window is presumably sufficiently elastic to allow the fluid of these canals to move in sympathy with movements of the oval window. Since most of the membranous labyrinth is relatively incompressible these perilymphatic movements could lead to displacements of the tectorial membrane relative to the basilar membrane, especially if the latter is the more elastic of the two membranes. This could lead to stimulation of the auditory receptors on the

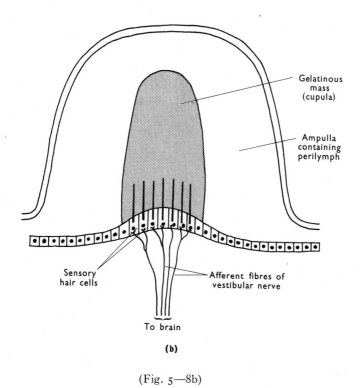

(Fig. 5—8b)

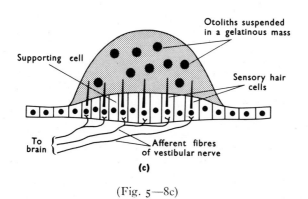

(Fig. 5—8c)

basilar membrane. The basilar membrane gets progressively broader and thicker as it proceeds towards the apex of the cochlea. According to direct microscopic observations the vibrations of the basilar membrane are maximal near the apex of the cochlea for high frequency sounds and maximal near the base for low frequencies. It seems likely, therefore, that the sensory receptors on different parts of the basilar membrane are activated by different sound frequencies and in this manner the brain is able to determine the tone, quality and loudness of the sound collected by the external ears. The mammalian cochlea is evidently designed to present the brain with details of the component frequencies of very complex sounds.

The mammalian cochlea has its origin in the lagena of lower vertebrates. The lagena is a sac-like prominence of the membranous labyrinth. It is rudimentary in fishes and amphibians but takes on certain characteristics of the mammalian cochlea in reptiles and birds (Fig. 5–9). The middle ear first appears in anuran amphibians, such as frogs and toads, where it consists of an air-filled pouch which separates the outer wall of the auditory capsule, containing the inner ear, from the skin (Fig. 5–10). The outer wall of the middle ear is fused to the skin to form a membrane, the tympanum

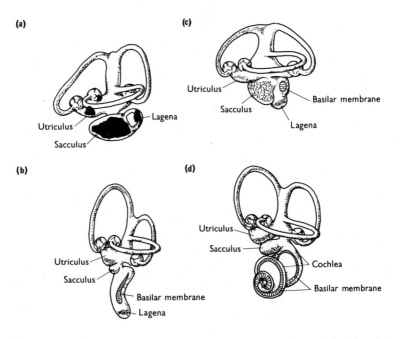

**Fig. 5–9**  Membranous labyrinths of various vertebrates. (a) fish; (b) reptile; (c) bird; (d) mammal. (From VON FRISCH, 1936.)

or ear drum, which is visible externally as a more or less circular patch on
the side of the head, just behind the eye (Plate 6). A slender bone, the
columella auris is attached to the inner surface of the tympanic membrane.
This bone, which presumably serves a similar function to the ossicles of
the mammalian middle ear, bridges the cavity of the middle ear and
articulates with a small bone, the stapes. The latter abuts onto an oval membrane, the fenestra ovalis, in the wall of the inner ear (Fig. 5–10).

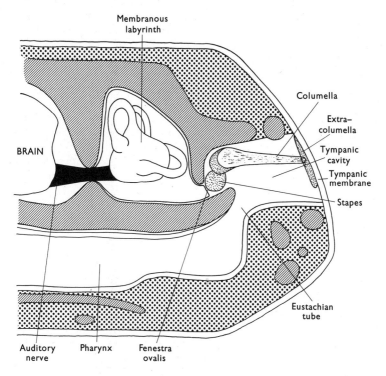

**Fig. 5–10**   Transverse section of the head of a frog illustrating the auditory
apparatus. Skeletal structures with the exception of the columella and stapes
are cross-hatched. (After PARKER & HASWELL, 1951.)

In general, as one ascends the phylogenetic scale, the complexity and
flexibility of the vertebrate hearing apparatus increases. This is not
particularly obvious, however, if one just compares the frequency sensitivities of different vertebrate ears. The human ear is most sensitive to
auditory stimuli in the range from 800 Hz–8500 Hz, with an upper limit
around 16 000 Hz (Fig. 5–11). The cartilaginous fishes, which have
auditory receptors in the sacculus and utriculus, respond to sound frequencies up to 750 Hz, while in bony fishes, where the sacculus and lagena are

involved in hearing, sensitivity to 13 000 Hz has been noted. In reptiles where the auditory receptors are in the lagena, the frequency range is 5–10 000 Hz. In birds, which also use the lagena for auditory reception, the range extends to 25 000 Hz. The auditory system of the bat is one of the most highly specialized amongst the vertebrates. It is sensitive to frequencies up to 100 kHz. Although the visual part of the bat brain is poorly developed this animal is a good flier. Indeed the minor significance of vision in bats is indicated by the fact that these animals can navigate in complete darkness, provided that they can receive auditory information from their surroundings. Recent studies have shown that they use a form of echo-location to navigate their surroundings and to hunt for their prey. They emit very high frequency (up to 100 kHz) sound pulses which are well above the range of human hearing and interpret their surroundings on the basis of echoes that they receive. It might seem reasonable to assume that the prey of bats would be helpless in avoiding attacks from such formidable opponents, i.e. opponents that can be neither seen nor heard. However, a group of moths and lacewings commonly hunted by bats can detect the ultrasonic pulses emitted by their predators and are able to take avoiding action during an attack. Cetaceans (e.g. dolphins) also generate high frequency (20–200 kHz) sounds and use these acoustic signals, which are in the form of 'clicks', for echo-location.

The ears of moths and many other insects consist of tympanal organs located either on legs, thorax or abdomen. The tympanal organ consists of

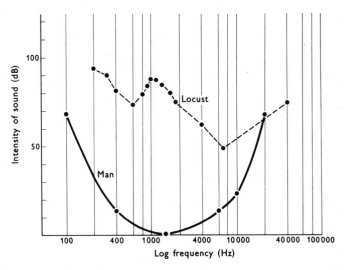

**Fig. 5-11** Comparison of threshold intensity of tympanal organ of the locust, *Schistocerca gregaria* and of man for pure tone sounds (Modified after UVAROV, 1966.)

an ear drum or tympanum to which a number of sensory neurons are
attached, processes from these auditory neurons sometimes being embedded in the tympanic membrane. When the membrane vibrates in response
to sound waves impinging upon it, the sensory neurons are excited. The
locusts have a tympanal organ on each side of the first abdominal segment
(Plate 7). It consists of a sclerotized ring forming a recess in the abdomen,
encircling a bean shaped tympanum (Fig. 5–12). The locust tympanal

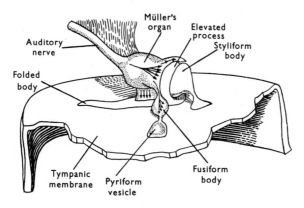

**Fig. 5–12**  Anatomy of the tympanal organ of the locust, *Locusta migratoria*.
Four groups of sensory receptors are located within Müller's organ, the
arrows indicating the direction of their dendrites. (From UVAROV; 1966;
redrawn after GRAY, 1960.)

organ contains 60–80 sensory neurons arranged in four groups and
attached to modified parts of the tympanum, the attachment points being
thickened regions of the tympanic membrane. The maximum sensitivity of
each group of receptor cells is limited to a small number of discrete frequency bands, ranging from 1·5 Hz for some cells to 19 Hz for others.
By having many auditory neurons with different peak sensitivities, a locust
can obtain a considerable amount of information about auditory stimuli
arriving at the ear drum (Fig. 5–11). In general, however, the hearing
apparatus of insects is rather limited in function. It is clearly tuned to
receive particular sounds but has little flexibility to deal with other types of
accoustic signal.

5.2.2.  EQUILIBRIUM RECEPTORS

The equilibrium and auditory senses are closely associated in most
vertebrates and invertebrates and the same sensory structure frequently
performs both functions. For instance, statocyst receptors (statoreceptors)
found in many invertebrates, often respond to vibrations as well as functioning as position receptors and receptors for linear and angular

(rotational) accelerations. They invariably consist of sensory hair cells which are acted upon by movements of a dense particle(s), the statolith suspended in a fluid of lower density than that of the statolith. In crayfish and lobsters the statocyst consists of a hollow cavity formed by invagination of the cuticle in the dorsal region of the basal joint of the antennule (Fig. 5–13a) and, as such, it is part of the external environment. The statocyst cavity contains a crescent shaped mass of about 400 sensory cells with hairs that are arranged in four rows (Fig. 5–13b). The three innermost rows of hairs are in contact with the statolith mass, which in these animals is often composed of sand grains introduced into the statocyst cavity during moulting. The hair cells act as position detectors, different groups of hairs being excited for each angular position of the antennule segment. The afferent fibres from the sensory hair cells continuously transmit information to the brain in the form of action potentials but when acted upon by the statolith their firing frequency changes. It is the directional displacement of the sensory hairs, or the shearing force exerted upon them by the statolith mass that excites the sensory receptors and not the downward or vertical pressure exerted by the statolith on the hairs. Other sensory hair cells found in the statocyst cavity are not attached to the statolith and are not excited by the changes in its position (Fig. 5–13b). These cells are excited by movements of the fluid in the statocyst cavity and are, therefore, receptors for rotational accelerations.

In many animals equilibrium receptors are important for reflex maintenance of muscle tone and body posture. The statocyst reflexes of crayfish and lobster, which are used for this purpose, can be examined by using the simple apparatus illustrated in Fig. 5–14. The positions of eyes and legs of

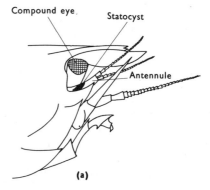

Compound eye    Statocyst

Antennule

(a)

**Fig. 5–13**   (a) Head of the crayfish, *Astacus*, illustrating position of statocyst receptor in basal joint of antennule. (b) Diagrammatic representation of the statolith and sensory hairs of the statocyst receptor. Afferent fibres from the sensory hair cells travel to the crayfish brain along the pathway indicated by the arrow.

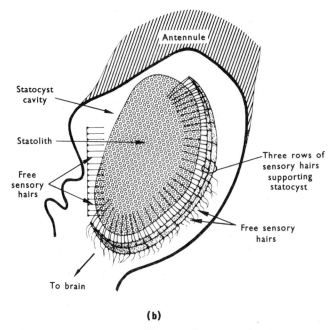

**(b)**

Fig. 5–13b

one of these animals should be noted as the animal is rotated to the right and left or rotated around an anterior-posterior axis. At each position of the animal the number of degrees departure from its normal position should also be noted. The role of the statocysts in the antennules in determining the positions of legs and eyes can be investigated by repeating the experiment with either one or both of the statocysts removed. In order to obtain the best results from this experiment it is advisable to avoid intense directional illumination.

Equilibrium receptors not unlike those found in the crustacean statocyst are present in the utriculus, sacculus and semicircular canals of the vertebrate membranous labyrinth (Figs. 5–6, 5–8b–c). The semicircular canals sit on top of the utriculus and occupy three separate planes at right angles to one another, two vertical and one horizontal. At one end of each canal, at their junctions with the utriculus, there is an ampulla containing hair cells which act as sensory receptors for rotational accelerations. The sensory receptors are grouped in cristae and their sensory hairs are embedded in gelatinous structures called cupulae (Fig. 5–8b). Acceleration or deceleration in the plane of a canal results in movement of the endolymph contained within the canal and this moves the cupula. This produces a shearing force which causes deformation and excitation of the hair cells.

The utriculus and sacculus, and in fish the lagena also, contain sensory

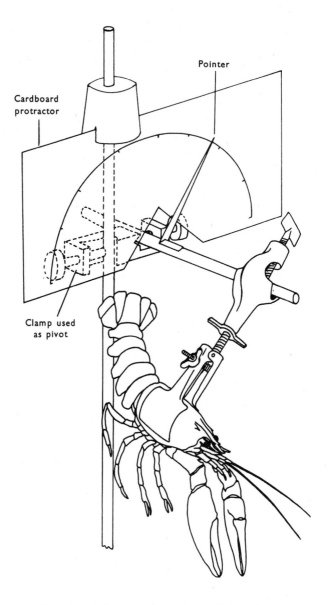

**Fig. 5–14** Experimental arrangement for studying the statocyst reflexes of the crayfish in response to tipping. (From WELSH, SMITH & KAMMER, 1968.) See text for further explanation.

receptors for measuring linear accelerations and position. These receptors consist of clusters of sensory hair cells arranged on plates called maculae (Fig. 5–8c). Each chamber usually contains more than one macula. The hairs of the sensory receptor cells are embedded in a gelatinous mass, containing high-density particles, called an otolith. Stimulation of the sensory receptors of the maculae occurs when the otolith acts tangentially on the hair cells.

## 5.3   Photoreception

Only a small part of the electromagnetic spectrum is visible light in human terms, the human visible spectrum ranging from about 38 nm (violet) to about 76 nm (red). Some animals respond to shorter wavelengths than those 'seen' by humans (ultraviolet) while others respond to longer wavelengths (infrared). Specialized sensory receptors, called photoreceptors, have been set aside to collect light energy. These cells endow an organism with the ability to measure the intensity, wavelength and directional properties of light. In lower animals the photoreceptors occur either singly or in small groups. In the latter case, they may form primitive eyes. In higher animals the photoreceptors are almost invariably associated with accessory structures with which they form sense organs, i.e. image-forming eyes.

### 5.3.1   THE ARTHROPOD COMPOUND EYE

The compound nature of the arthropod eye is readily apparent when its surface is viewed with a hand lens (Plate 8). It consists of an array of facets each of which may be flat or curved, sculptured or smooth and each of which represents the outer margin of a complete visual unit called an ommatidium (Fig. 5–15). The ommatidium is also the anatomical unit of the compound eye and comprises a cuticular lens, a refractile transparent crystalline cone which concentrates light entering the ommatidium into a narrow beam, and seven or eight elongated sensory cells, the retinula (retinal) cells (Fig. 5–16). The lens and crystalline cone jointly comprise the lens of the ommatidium and since the optical properties of these two structures are fixed, it follows that the focal length of the ommatidium is also fixed. The retinula cells are primary sensory cells and they make up the retina of the arthropod compound eye. Along their long axes, the inner margins (rhabdomes) of the retinula cells contribute to a region of high refractive index, the rhabdom, and it is this region of the ommatidium that absorbs light energy and presumably transduces it to electrical energy. In some compound eyes the rhabdom makes direct contact with the crystalline cone, but in others the retinula cells lie some distance from the crystalline cone and are connected to it by a transparent thread of material of high refractive index, called the crystalline tract. In many insects each omma-tidium is surrounded by two groups of pigment cells. A proximal group of

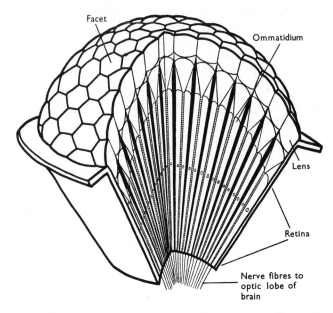

Facet

Ommatidium

Lens

Retina

Nerve fibres to
optic lobe of
brain

**Fig. 5–15** Diagrammatic representation of the compound eye of an insect illustrating the arrangement of the ommatidia. (From BUCHSBAUM, 1948.)

pigment cells encircles the retinula cells and, sometimes, also a group of distal pigment cells that ensheath the crystalline cone (Fig. 5–16a). In crustaceans the pigment is contained either wholly within the retinula cells, or within these cells as well as within a distal group of pigment cells (Fig. 5–16b). In eyes where the retinula cells make direct contact with the crystalline cone, the pigment cells are more or less fixed in position and effectively isolate each ommatidium from its neighbours. These so-called apposition eyes are found in arthropods that live in high light intensities. Insects such as moths and crustaceans such as lobsters, which live in low light intensities, have so-called superposition eyes, in which the pigment migrates up and down the long axis of the ommatidium with changes in light intensity. In bright light the ommatidia of superposition eyes are effectively isolated from each other by the pigment, but in weak light the pigment cells retract. Apparently this mechanism protects the eyes from high light intensities rather than improving the light trapping ability of the eye when it is exposed to dim light by allowing light to cross ommatidia as was formerly imagined. The crystalline tract which connects the crystalline cone and rhabdom possibly acts as a lightguide retaining and conducting light by internal reflection. In bright light the pigment covers the tract and reduces internal reflection and as a result the amount of light reaching the retinula cells is also reduced.

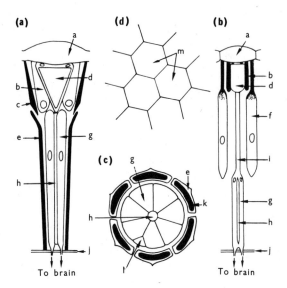

**Fig. 5–16** (a) Ommatidium from compound eye of an arthropod living in high light intensities. (b) Ommatidium from compound eye of an arthropod living in low light intensities. (c) Transverse section of (a) at level of retinula cells. (d) Hexagonal arrangement of ommatidia seen from surface of eye. (After WIGGLESWORTH, 1965.)

a, corneal lens; b, matrix cells of cornea; c, primary pigment cells; d, crystalline cone; e, secondary pigment cells; f, pigment cell; g, retinula cells; h, rhabdom; i, crystaline tract; j, fenestrated basement membrane; k, pigment; l, eccentric retinula cell; m, facets.

The compound eyes of arthropods can discriminate the intensity, direction, colour and the plane of polarization of light. The ability to distinguish colours is based upon differences in spectral sensitivity of different classes of retinula cells. Presumably these cells contain different classes of photochemical pigments (not to be confused with the 'protective' pigments), the retinula cells being depolarized when light of a particular wavelength range is absorbed by these pigments. In some compound eyes the retinula cells function as independent units and generate receptor potentials which activate their afferent fibres to produce action potentials. In a few arthropods the electrical information from the retinula cells, i.e. the receptor potentials, is first collected by an eccentric cell which lies amongst the sense cells and it is this eccentric cell which generates and transmits action potentials to the brain. It is of course important to remember that interpretation of information received by the eye is performed mainly by the brain, especially the optic lobes, and there is no evidence that the arthropod brain actually 'sees' the image which forms on the arthropod retina.

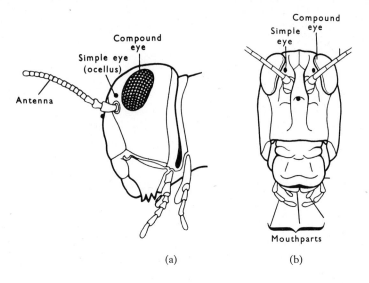

(a)                                        (b)

**Fig. 5–17**  Head of the locust viewed from the side (a) and from the front (b) showing position of simple eyes and compound eyes. (From BUCHSBAUM, 1948; after SNODGRASS, 1935.)

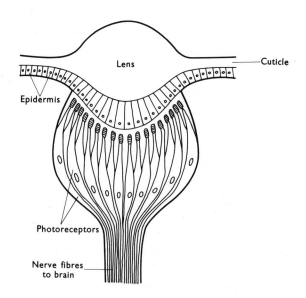

**Fig. 5–18**  Simple eye or ocellus of a spider. The photoreceptors share a single cuticular lens. (From BUCHSBAUM, 1948.)

Apart from compound eyes some arthropods also have less sophisticated eyes called ocelli (Fig. 5-17). These are found also in coelenterates, flatworms and annelids. Some ocelli form images but most respond only to light intensity (Fig. 5-18).

The most striking difference between vertebrate eyes and arthropod compound eyes seems to be that the visible part of the spectrum for the arthropod eye is shifted, relative to that of the vertebrate eye, 100 nm towards the shorter wavelengths, i.e. the arthropod eye has a pronounced ultraviolet sensitivity as well as a sensitivity in the part of the spectrum visible to humans.

### 5.3.2    THE VERTEBRATE EYE

The vertebrate eye is frequently compared with the photographic camera but in fact is more analogous to the television camera. Its function is to convey information about a changing visual field to the brain in the form of spatially and temporally arranged nerve impulse patterns. Unlike a photographic camera it does not fix an image. Any image that is stationary on the photosensitive surface of the eye is observed by the brain for only a very brief period. Fixed objects in the visual field can only be observed over long periods by moving the eyes so that the position of the image on the retina is constantly varied. Our eyes are continuously moving, even when we stare at an object!

The amount of light entering the eye is controlled by a reflex system involving the iris which acts like a camera diaphragm. The light passes through a series of refractive surfaces. It first crosses the transparent cornea and then passes through the aqueous humor. It then passes through the crystalline lens and vitreous humor before reaching the nervous layer of the eye and eventually the retina (Fig. 5-19). The image of an object in the visual field of the eye must be sharply focused on the retina if it is to be clearly 'seen' by the brain. Normally, the eye can adequately accommodate objects at different distances by changing the shape of the lens, and hence its focal length, by means of the ciliary muscles. In sufferers of myopia (short-sightedness) distant objects are focused in front of the retina. This is counteracted by placing a concave lens in front of the eye. In sufferers of hypermetropia (long-sightedness) objects are focused behind the retina and a convex lens is required to correct the fault. Sometimes the eye lens loses its elasticity and as a result objects close to the eye cannot be focused. This condition is called presbyopia and can be corrected by a convex lens. A few people suffer from a condition known as astigmatism, in which the corneal and lens surfaces are irregular and as a result there are spatial variations in focal length.

The retina is the photoreceptive part of the vertebrate eye. It is formed by an outgrowth of the brain (Fig. 5-20) and is composed of a thin layer of cells lining the back of the eyeball, the cells being of two different types, namely rods and cones. There are many tens of thousands of these receptors

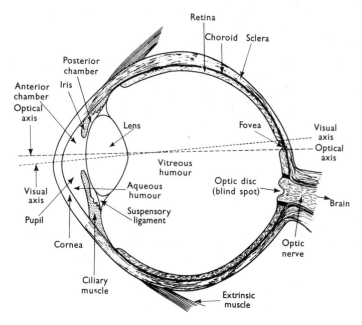

**Fig. 5–19** The human eye, an example of a complex sense organ. The orientation of the eyeball in the eye socket is controlled by six sets of muscles (not all shown) controlled by three pairs of nerves. The receptive area of the eye is the retina, the innermost layer of the external covering of the eyeball. Accessory non-receptive structures are important optically: the iris acts as a light diaphragm: the lens and associated ciliary muscles enable the eye to focus images of objects located at different distances from the eye. (After MAXIMOV & BLOOM, 1957 *Textbook of Histology*. W. B. Saunders, Philadelphia.)

in each square millimetre of retina and as a result the resolving powers of the vertebrate eye are immensely superior to those of the arthropod compound eye. The rods and cones are primary sensory units and their ratio varies according to the mode of life of the animal. Nocturnal animals usually have more rods than cones and may also have, in addition, a reflective surface called a tapetum which reflects light back into the eye after it has passed through the retina. The eyes of some diurnal animals may contain more cones than rods and in some diurnal animals (e.g. owls) rods may be absent altogether.

In terms of neural organisation the retina contains five types of nerve cell; photoreceptors, i.e. the rods and cones, bipolar neurons, amacrine neurons, horizontal neurons and ganglion cells. The bipolar neurons and ganglion cells provide pathways from the photoreceptors to the brain and they are connected laterally by the amacrine cells. The horizontal cells

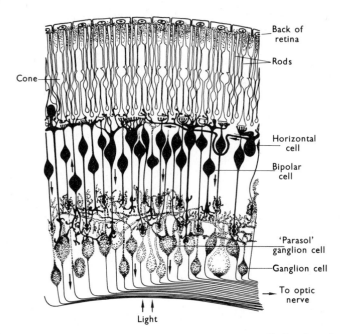

Back of
retina

Rods

Cone

Horizontal
cell

Bipolar
cell

'Parasol'
ganglion cell

Ganglion cell

To optic
nerve

Light

Fig. 5–20   The human retina. The photoreceptors are called rods and cones
and they lie at the base of the retina. To reach them light must pass through
two layers of neurons which are involved in integrating information collected
by the photoreceptors and transferring the processed data to the brain
through the optic nerve. Some of the connections between the afferent pathways involve inhibitory synapses which can attenuate or even switch off the
output of a sensory unit. Direction of information flow indicated by arrows.
(From GREGORY, 1966.)

form lateral pathways between the rods and cones. The vertebrate retina
is inverted, so that the tips of the rods and cones point towards the back of
the eyeball rather than towards the lens. Afferent fibres from the ganglion
cells pass across the inner face of the retina and enter the optic nerve. There
are no rods and cones in the region where the optic nerve pierces the retina
and leaves the eyeball. This region is aptly called the blind-spot. In man,
fibres from the outer side of the retina pass to the optic centre on the same
side of the brain, but those from the inner (nasal) side of the retina cross
over just behind the eyes, at the optic chiasma, and go to the opposite side
of the brain. It is in this complex wiring pattern that the properties of three-
dimensional vision reside.

Electrical potentials are generated in the rods and cones when the photosensitive pigments that they contain absorb light energy. We cannot
experience the reception of individual quanta of light by one of our eyes

(5–8 quanta are required to give the *experience* of a flash of light) but the photoreceptors are so sensitive that they can be excited by a single quantum. The best-known visual pigments are the visual purples which occur in the rods receptors and in the photoreceptors of many invertebrates. These consist of a carotenoid chromophore, retinene and a protein, opsin. The visual purple of the rod receptor is called rhodopsin. It is reddish in colour and absorbs light in the yellow-green part of the visual spectrum, i.e. about 500 nm. When it is exposed to light rhodopsin is bleached to retinene, the aldehyde of vitamin A, and opsin and in some unknown way this reaction leads to the production of a receptor potential across the membrane of the rod receptor. Cone receptors do not contain rhodopsin, but may contain another pigment called iodopsin, which consists of a retinene plus cone opsin (photopsin). In man the cones are responsible for colour vision and it is likely that there are three different types of cone, each type containing one of three different pigments, sensitive to red, green and blue respectively. The other colours of the visual spectrum can be produced by appropriate mixing of these three colours.

### 5.4 Optokinesis

The majority of animals which possess eyes either move their eyes or other parts of their bodies or even their whole bodies when confronted by a changing visual field. These movements are called optokinetic responses and they can be readily investigated in crustaceans and insects by rotating a cylinder with vertical black and white stripes around these animals (Plate 9). Insects such as flies and locusts can be used to demonstrate optokinetic responses by placing them on a stationary platform suspended in the centre of such a cylinder. The floor of the cylinder and platform should be lined with white paper and the inside of the cylinder should be evenly illuminated. By mounting the cylinder on the shaft of a kymograph it can be smoothly rotated at different speeds. Usually, the insect will turn in the same direction as the stripes are moved, but at a slower rate when the cylinder is revolved very slowly, the insect will not turn, but may still move its head (the eyes cannot move on their own) in the direction that the stripes are moving and then flick it back to its initial position before resuming its tracking of the stripes. This sort of behaviour is called optokinetic nystagmus. The posture of the insect may also change as the cylinder is rotated with the insect showing a tendency to lean in the direction of movement of the stripes. In crustaceans such as crabs, in which the eyes are on stalks or eyecups, movements of the eyes occur in response to a changing visual field. If a crab is held by a clamp in the centre of a revolving striped cylinder the eyes undergo optokinetic nystagmus.

Experiments of this type have been used to investigate many different properties of compound eyes. For example, the acuity of the eye can be examined by using striped cylinders with different stripe widths and colour vision can be tested for by using stripes of different colours but equal brightness. It is also possible to demonstrate that crabs and locusts store information about their visual field. If a crab is used it is suspended in a stationary cylinder which is illuminated for a few minutes. It is then plunged into complete darkness and the cylinder is turned through a small angle. Under these conditions the crab's eyes do not move. But if the cylinder is re-illuminated after a short period of time the crab's eyes move in the same direction as the cylinder was moved. Apparently the crab remembers the former position of the image of the striped drum on its retina and notes that it does not correspond with the new position of the image. As a result it takes the appropriate action to restore the original image position.

The functional significance of optokinetic responses in arthropods remains somewhat obscure. Undoubtedly movement of eyes and head sharpen up vision but there is no evidence that the arthropod can 'see' only moving objects. There is evidence, however, that optokinetic responses are the basis for compass reactions to the sun that occur in some crustaceans. For example, in the absence of any landmarks except the sun, some littoral amphipods are able to head correctly towards the sea when too dry or towards land when submerged. Apparently the position of the sun at different times of the day is taken into account by reference to an internal rhythm within these animals. When the shore crab, *Carcinus*, is dropped onto a surface without landmarks it requires only 10 seconds before it shows a demonstrable response to the movement of the sun.

In theory all vertebrates should be able to move their two eyes independently, and in lower vertebrates this frequently happens. In man, voluntary movements of the eyes are normally co-ordinated in such a manner that the same part of an object is always focused simultaneously on the two foveas, i.e. the retinal regions containing the highest population density of rods.

# Integrative Properties of
# Nervous Systems 6

The behaviour of an animal is influenced and, indeed, often determined by the information that it receives from sensory receptors that may well be distributed all over its body. It is the function of a nervous system to collect and process this information and to control the appropriate reaction to it. In other words, the integrative action of a nervous system is to transfer diverse and even conflicting sensory messages into a unified course of motor events.

## 6.1 Integration at synapses

The synaptic connections between excitable cells are the site of much integrative activity, since synaptic potentials and receptor potentials are usually graded, rather than all-or-nothing, electrical events and can therefore interact and recombine, over and over again, in space and time. Even a single synapse may contribute some measure of integration through summation and facilitation of synaptic potentials. At some excitatory synapses, such as those on phasic striated muscle fibres in vertebrates, an action potential in the presynaptic neuron always initiates an action potential in the postsynaptic element (transmission is 1:1) and there is, therefore, no obvious integration. However, if the EPSP's are normally subthreshold events, as is frequently the case at many central synapses, then action potentials will appear in the postsynaptic cell only

**Fig. 6–1** Temporal summation (b) and facilitation (c). A neuron, the presynaptic cell, makes an excitatory synapse with another neuron, the postsynaptic cell. When an action potential arrives at the terminal of the presynaptic cell a depolarizing excitatory postsynaptic potential (EPSP) appears in the postsynaptic cell. The synaptic response is insufficient to evoke an action potential in the spike-generating membrane of this cell (a). However, if two impulses arrive in close succession at the presynaptic terminal then the two resultant EPSP's summate and depolarization of the postsynaptic cell now exceeds the threshold for generation of an action potential (b). This process is called temporal summation. The excitatory postsynaptic potential also increases in magnitude with repetition and in (c), where the frequency of the presynaptpic impulses is lower than it is in (b), the third EPSP is sufficiently large to evoke an action potential, even though there is no summation. This growth of the synaptic potential with repetition is called facilitation. In (a–c), the top traces represent the action potentials recorded from the presynaptic terminal, while the bottom traces represent recordings from the postsynaptic cell.

after temporal summation and/or facilitation of the EPSP's (Fig. 6–1). During summation excitatory EPSP's add more or less arithmetically, while during facilitation the synaptic potentials grow in magnitude with repetition. At some synapses the magnitude of the synaptic potential declines with repetition. This is called synaptic fatigue or depression. At excitatory synapses synaptic fatigue can result in the transformation of a suprathreshold EPSP, i.e. one which will initiate an action potential in the postsynaptic cell, to a subthreshold event. Temporal summation, facilitation and synaptic fatigue also occur at inhibitory synapses.

When a postsynaptic cell receives convergent inputs then the possibilities for integration are considerable (Fig. 6–2). This can occur through temporal and spatial summation of synaptic potentials, through facilitation at individual synapses (homolateral facilitation), and possibly also through a second type of facilitation in which activity at one synapse facilitates the

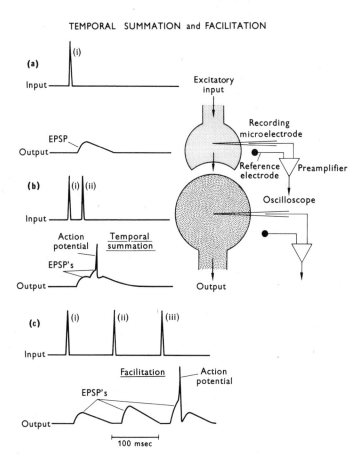

TEMPORAL SUMMATION and FACILITATION

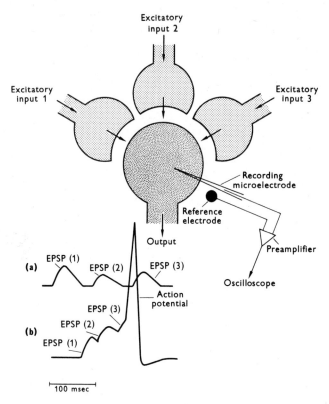

**Fig. 6–2** Spatial summation of synaptic events. A single neuron, the postsynaptic cell, forms excitatory synapses with three presynaptic neurons. Stimulation of any one of these presynaptic neurons produces an EPSP which is insufficient to evoke an action potential in the postsynaptic cell (a). However, when the three presynaptic inputs are stimulated in quick succession the resultant EPSP's summate and the depolarization of the postsynaptic cell is now sufficient to trigger the production of an action potential (b).

synaptic events at adjacent synapses (heterolateral facilitation). Integration at the synaptic level becomes more complex when a neuron has excitatory and inhibitory inputs, since the inhibitory postsynaptic potentials (IPSP's) and EPSP's sum algebraically (Fig. 6–3). The possibilities for integration are further increased by presynaptic inhibition (and possibly also presynaptic excitation) (Fig. 6–4). The important point to remember is that a postsynaptic element can handle any number of subthreshold events, so long as its membrane potential does not exceed the threshold level for spike initiation.

Thorax

Compound eye
with ommatidia

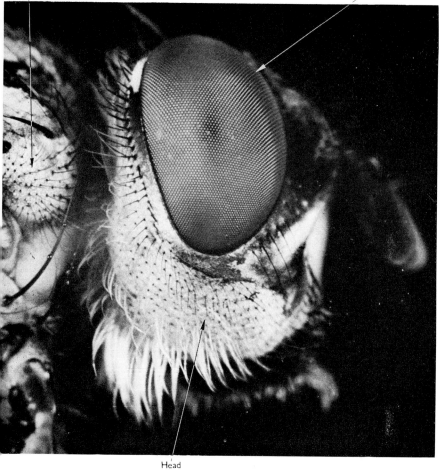

Head

**Plate 8**  Side view of the head and anterior thorax of a blowfly (*Sarcophaga barbata*) showing position of the compound eye and surface view of the ommatidia of which it is composed.

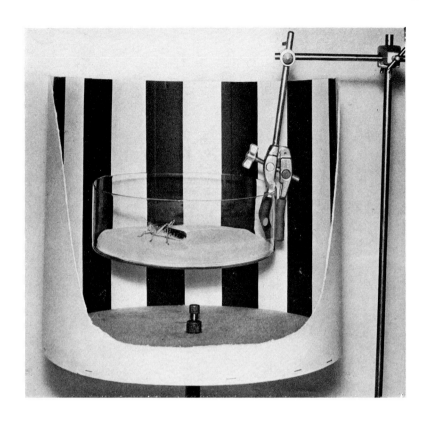

**Plate 9**  Photograph of experimental arrangement for studying optokinetic responses of animals. A locust has been placed in a large crystallizing dish which is suspended by a clamp in the centre of a striped cylinder (partly removed). The cylinder is made of cardboard and is attached to a circular wooden plate, which is, in turn, attached to the shaft of a kymograph. See text for further details.

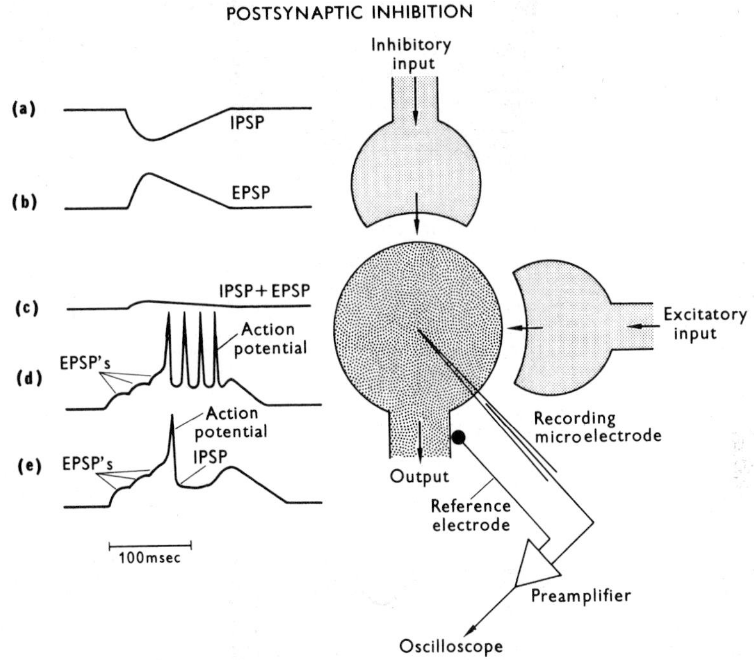

**Fig. 6-3** Postsynaptic inhibition. A neuron, the postsynaptic cell, synapses with the terminals of two other neurons, the presynaptic cells. Stimulation of one of the presynaptic neurons, i.e. the excitatory input, evokes a subthreshold depolarizing EPSP in the postsynaptic cell (b). Repetitive stimulation of this presynaptic neuron evokes a train of EPSP's which summate and facilitate and are accompanied by action potentials (d). Stimulation of the other presynaptic cell, i.e. the inhibitory input, evokes a hyperpolarizing inhibitory postsynaptic potential (IPSP) (a). When both presynaptic neurons are excited, the EPSP and IPSP that they set up in the post-synaptic cell sum algebraically (c), and when an IPSP occurs during a train of EPSP's generation of action potentials by the postsynaptic neuron is inhibited during the IPSP (e).

The spatial arrangement of synapses on central neurons is of considerable importance in influencing the level of integration. Usually the membrane at the axon hillock has by far the lowest critical depolarization threshold and is therefore the initiating site for action potentials. If the synapses are some distance from this site, for example if they are on the dendrites, then there is more scope for integration. This is because synaptic potentials will probably be very subthreshold at the spike initiating zone, since they spread decrementally. This means that currents generated at excitatory synapses will be much more effective in influencing the generation of action potentials by the postsynaptic cell if these synapses are situated

PRESYNAPTIC INHIBITION

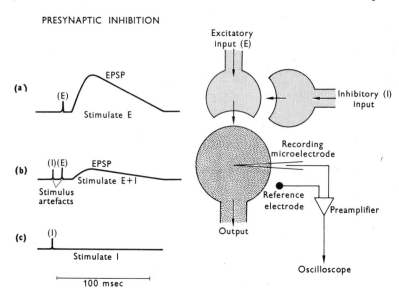

**Fig. 6–4** Presynaptic inhibition. A neuron, the postsynaptic cell, synapses with an excitatory neuron (E), the presynaptic cell. The terminal of the excitatory neuron also makes contact with the terminal of a second presynaptic neuron, which is inhibitory (I). Stimulation of the excitatory presynaptic neuron produces a large EPSP in the postsynaptic cell (a). However, when an action potential reaches the terminal of the inhibitory presynaptic neuron just prior to the arrival of an action potential at the terminal, the excitatory presynaptic neuron transmission at the excitatory synapse is either partly inhibited (b) or completely repressed. Stimulation of the inhibitory presynaptic neuron alone does not evoke a response from the postsynaptic neuron (c).

close to the axon hillock. Similarly currents generated at inhibitory synapses will be most effective in preventing spike formation if these inhibitory synapses are positioned near the spike initiating zone, or if the inhibitory synapses are interposed between the axon hillock and the excitatory synapses. Perhaps this is the reason why inhibitory synapses are frequently found on the somata or axons of many vertebrate central neurons, where they will be most effective in switching off the output of the cell, whilst the excitatory synapses are restricted to the dendrites. The most important point to remember is that when a neuron has many hundreds of both excitatory and inhibitory inputs, producing synaptic potentials of different magnitudes, a remarkably high level of integration can be achieved by discrete positioning of the synapses and by spatially organizing them in relation to the spike generating site of the postsynaptic cell. Integrative activity is not limited, of course, to synapses. The non-synaptic membrane of the postsynaptic cell can also perform an integrative function through adaptation or accommodation of its spike generation mechanism and through refractoriness.

In arthropods some integrative activity occurs at synapses between motor neurons and muscle fibres. In these animals a single muscle fibre may be innervated by one or more excitatory motor neurons as well as one or more inhibitory motor neurons, the excitatory and inhibitory synapses being distributed at intervals along the entire length of the fibre. (Fig. 4.3). The non-synaptic membrane of most arthropod muscle fibres generates electrical responses of variable amplitude, rather than all-or-none action potentials, when it is depolarized by currents associated with the appearance of suprathreshold EPSP's at the excitatory synapses. Spatial and temporal summation of EPSP's and IPSP's together with synaptic fatigue, facilitation and presynaptic inhibition at the synaptic sites and refractoriness of the non-synaptic membrane of arthropod muscle fibres, account for the high level of peripheral integrative activity in this system. By placing an integrative zone in its peripheral nervous system, the arthropod is able to exert very fine control over the muscle fibres and economize on the number of motor neurons that are needed for this purpose. This is of great value to animals with limited space in their central nervous systems. Such economy is not so essential in vertebrates and here the main method of grading the force developed by a skeletal muscle is to divide the muscle into units, called motor units, each unit containing a group of muscle fibres innervated by a single motor neuron. A muscle may contain many hundreds of these motor units and the force that it develops can be graded by varying the number of motor units active at any one time, a process which is termed recruitment. Some vertebrate tonic muscle fibres are multiterminally and polyneuronally innervated. These cannot produce action potentials and function in much the same way as arthropod skeletal muscle fibres.

## 6.2 Nerve nets

A diffuse randomly organized network of nerve cells is perhaps the simplest possible assemblage of interacting neurons. This type of organization is exemplified by the coelenterate nerve net which may well represent the simplest type of nervous system in the animal kingdom. Nevertheless, the coelenterate nerve net is a very complex assemblage of interacting units and the site of much integrative activity. Because coelenterates have diffuse nervous conduction systems, many of their motor activities are quite local and do not usually involve the whole organism. Indeed even isolated parts of a coelenterate appear to behave quite normally (Fig. 6–5). In corals and other colonial coelenterates the individual members of the colony are joined together by a nerve net. In some corals the nerve net contains through-conduction pathways, and stimulation of part of a

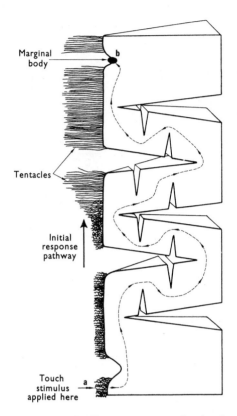

**Fig. 6–5** Demonstration of diffuse nervous conduction involving two conduction systems in the jellyfish, *Aurelia*. A part of the edge of the bell of a jellyfish was isolated and cut as shown in the diagram. When all the tentacles were fully relaxed, region **a** was stimulated mechanically (with a pinch). The stimulus was followed by a wave of tentacle contraction which spread along the edge of the bell. Due to the cuts in the bell it follows that conduction of information which resulted in tentacle contraction followed a pathway around the cuts indicated by the dotted line and arrows. When this information reached the ganglion at **b**, it initiated a wave of contraction of the bell musculature which spread back to **a**. Although the information which travelled from **b** to **a** and which resulted in tentacle contraction, followed the same route overall as the information, which travelled from **a** to **b** and which resulted in contraction of the bell musculature, the former travelled at half the speed of the latter. Because the two waves of information had different conduction velocities and caused different responses, this is strong circumstantial evidence for the existence of two nerve nets. (After HORRIDGE, 1968.)

colony evokes maximal contractions from all members of the colony. In other colonial hydroids, where the nerve net is less highly organized, the size of the responding area usually increases with increasing number of stimuli and with increasing stimulus strength (Fig. 6–6). The response is graded in this manner because the synapses between neurons of the nerve net, and possibly also synapses on the effectors, must be facilitated before action potentials in a presynaptic cell will generate suprathreshold EPSP's in postsynaptic cell. In other words, a number of action potentials must arrive at the terminals of the presynaptic element in quick succession before an action potential will occur in the postsynaptic element. As a result, the number of action potentials travelling through a diffuse nerve net declines progressively as more and more synapses are crossed, since at each synapse the first few impulses in a train will fail to cross the synaptic cleft. The decline in number of nerve impulses with distance will

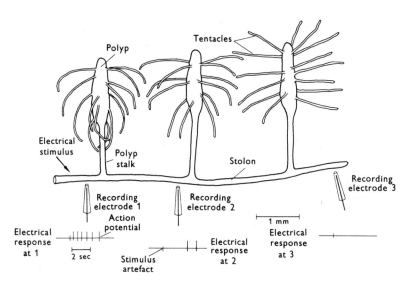

**Fig. 6–6**  A stimulus (electrical) was applied to the stolon of a colonial coelenterate (*Cordylophora*) at the point marked by the arrow. The polyp nearest the point of stimulation responded most to the stimulus, the next polyp responded slightly less, while the most distal polyp did not respond at all. This coelenterate has a local nerve net system and the responses of this animal therefore decline in magnitude with distance from a stimulated site. Recordings of the electrical activity at different points in this nerve net demonstrated a long burst of nerve impulses at the stalk of the nearest polyp, a shorter burst at the stalk of the next polyp, whereas at the stalk of the distal polyp no potentials were recorded following the stimulus. (After JOSEPHSON, 1961 )

be associated with a decline in the magnitude of the muscle contraction
with distance from the stimulated site.

## 6.3   Reflexes and nervous integration

When the nervous system is viewed as a whole the reflex may be considered as the basic unit of nervous integration. Anatomically a reflex
consists, in its simplest form, of an afferent neuron linked either directly to
an effector, as is possibly the case in some coelenterates, or indirectly
through a motor neuron. Many leg reflexes in arthropods possibly involve
only afferent and efferent neurons and in humans the knee jerk reflex is a
good example of a simple reflex involving only two sets of neurons. Nor-

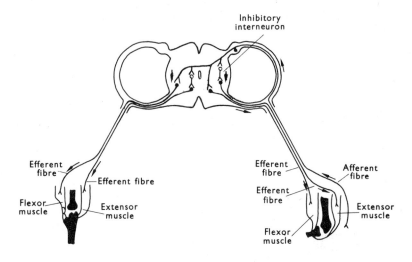

**Fig. 6–7**   Reciprocal innervation and cross reflexes in man. The alternating
contractions of flexor muscles and extensor muscles in the thigh which occur,
for example, during walking, are co-ordinated by reflex pathways involving
excitation and inhibition of motor neurons which innervate these muscles.
When the flexor muscles on the right side are activated they stretch the
extensor muscles of that side. This affects the output of the muscle spindles
and tendon organs associated with the extensor muscles. Impulses from these
sensory receptors pass along afferents to the spinal cord. The afferent fibres
communicate with extensor and flexor motor neurons of the right side, either
directly or through interneurons. They inhibit the flexor motor neurons and
excite the extensor motor neurons. As a result the flexor muscles relax and
the extensor muscles contract. The afferent fibres also cross to the left side
of the spinal cord and communicate with flexor and extensor motor neurons
of that side. However, on that side the flexor muscles are excited and contract
whilst the extensor motor neurons are inhibited and the extensor muscles
relax.

Reflex action

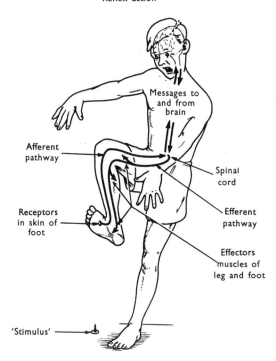

**Fig. 6–8**   It is important to remember that reflex actions, especially in more advanced animals, are very complex and may involve many nervous pathways. (From MCNAUGHT & CALLANDER, 1970.)

mally, however, when there is a well developed central nervous system excitatory and inhibitory interneurons are often interposed between the afferent and efferent neurons. In segmented animals intrasegmental interneurons connect afferent and efferent neurons of one side to form a segmental reflex pathway. These interneurons may also form cross reflex pathways, by connecting afferent neurons of one side with efferent neurons of the contralateral side (Fig. 6–7). Intersegmental interneurons, which connect afferent neurons of one segment to motor neurons of other segments and to neurons in the brain, also occur (Figs 6–8, 6–9), while a further set of interneurons may form connections between the brain and the segmental motor neurons (Fig. 6–10). Branches from afferent neurons may also course intersegmentally and in insects, at least, there is evidence that some motor neurons are intersegmental.

The control of posture is based upon information that streams into the nervous system from receptors distributed all over the body. Some of the

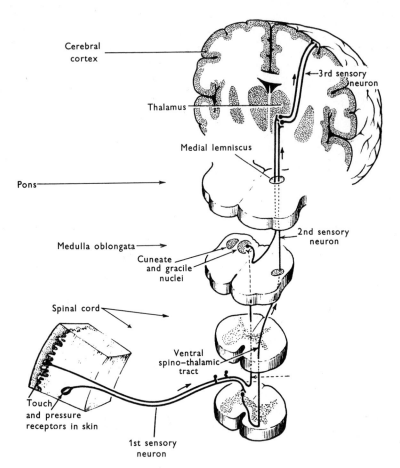

Cerebral cortex

3rd sensory neuron

Thalamus

Medial lemniscus

Pons

Medulla oblongata

2nd sensory neuron

Cuneate and gracile nuclei

Spinal cord

Ventral spino-thalamic tract

Touch and pressure receptors in skin

1st sensory neuron

**Fig. 6–9** Touch and pressure receptors in the mammalian trunk and limbs are connected by a chain of three neurons with the parietal lobes of the cerebral cortex. Processes of the 1st sensory neuron reach the gracile or cuneate nucleus of the medulla oblongata before synapsing with the 2nd sensory neuron. Other axon processes may just run up several segments of the spinal cord before synapsing with a 2nd sensory neuron or they may even terminate in their own segment of the cord. The processes of most of the 2nd sensory neurons cross the midline. (From McNAUGHT & CALLANDER, 1970.)

most important of these sensory structures are the mechanoreceptors associated with muscles and joints. In crustaceans muscle receptors or stretch receptors are found in most segments. For example, in the lobster tail there is a pair of muscle receptors in each segment on either side of the dorsal midline (Fig. 5–3). Each receptor pair contains a fast adapting receptor muscle and a slow adapting receptor muscle (Fig. 5–4). Each receptor consists of a muscle fibre which is suspended antero-posteriorly across a segment, and embedded in this muscle fibre are found the terminals or dendrites of a sensory neuron. When the muscle fibre is stretched during flexion of the tail the sensory dendrites are stimulated and a receptor potential is initiated. As a result, one or more action potentials may be generated in the sensory axon. Thus the muscle receptors provide for a continuous automatic feedback of information about the position of the tail. The muscle fibre and sensory neuron also receive information from the central nervous system of the lobster. This can produce useful variations in the sensitivity of the system. Inhibitory neurons, which innervate both the receptor muscle fibre and the sensory neuron, serve to reduce the sensitivity of the system by relaxing the muscle fibre and by attenuating the receptor potential. The excitatory motor neurons, which innervate the muscle fibre, increase the sensitivity of the system by causing the muscle fibre to contract, thereby generating a small receptor potential in the sensory neuron which sums with the receptor potential which occurs during flexion. The long-term output of the tonic or slow adapting receptor muscle reminds us that reflexes are not necessarily events of limited duration. Indeed, when a tonic sensory unit is coupled to a tonic motor unit reflex activity can occur over long periods.

Two main sets of sensory receptors, muscle stretch receptors and tendon receptors, are involved in the co-ordination of skeletal muscle activity in mammals. The stretch receptors consist of muscle fibres (intrafusal fibres) which are bundled together in a connective tissue capsule embedded in the skeletal muscles, and are connected in parallel with the main muscle fibres (extrafusal fibres) (Fig. 5–5). The intrafusal fibres carry endings from two types of sensory neurons, the annullospiral endings from 1A afferent neurons and the flower spray endings from 1B afferent neurons. The level of activity of the stretch receptors is controlled in part by the central nervous system through motor neurons, the gamma-motor neurons or gamma-efferents, which can alter the mechanical state of the intrafusal muscle fibres. When the extrafusal fibres contract in response to commands from alpha-motor neurons the stretch receptors are relaxed, and the discharges of the sensory neurons fall towards zero. When the extrafusal muscle fibres are stretched during contraction of an antagonistic muscle, the intrafusal fibres are also stretched and the action potentials generated by the sensory neurons increase in frequency. Stimulation of the gamma-efferents 'presets' the firing frequency of the sensory neurons of the stretch receptors and puts the system 'on alert'. The tendon receptors are sensory endings located in the tendons of the skeletal muscles and respond to tension changes in these muscles.

The flexion reflex, which represents the mechanism for withdrawing an extremity from injury, is the most primitive pattern of response of higher vertebrates. Motor neurons in many spinal segments are usually involved

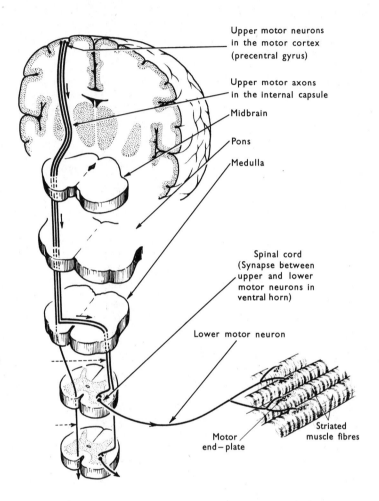

Upper motor neurons
in the motor cortex
(precentral gyrus)

Upper motor axons
in the internal capsule

Midbrain

Pons

Medulla

Spinal cord
(Synapse between
upper and lower
motor neurons in
ventral horn)

Lower motor neuron

Striated
muscle fibres

Motor
end–plate

**Fig. 6–10** Interneurons (sometimes called upper motor neurons) in the human motor cortex send axons through the brain which then usually cross over and run downwards in the lateral cortico-spinal tract, before synapsing with motor neurons (sometimes called lower motor neurons) in the ventral (anterior) horn of the spinal cord. The axons of the lower motor neurons travel in the spinal nerves to the skeletal muscles of the trunk and the limbs. Some of the axons of the upper motor neurons remain uncrossed and run down the spinal cord in the anterior cortico-spinal tract. (From MCNAUGHT & CALLANDER, 1970.)

simultaneously, e.g. all the flexor motor neurons of the hip, knee and ankle, and hence a single afferent nerve, which admittedly may contain many afferent neurons, nevertheless has the capacity to command many motor units. Mammalian extensor muscles are primarily concerned in resisting the action of gravity through the action of stretch reflexes. Reciprocal innervation of antagonistic extensor and flexor muscles ensures that when an extensor muscle contracts its opposing flexor muscle relaxes. This sort of activity involves central inhibition of flexor motor neurons through reflexly excited inhibitory interneurons (Fig. 6–7).

Most of the information entering the vertebrate spinal cord from the sensory systems of the body is communicated to the brain. The inter-neurons which connect afferent neurons with higher centres in the brain run in special tracts through the spinal cord and brain. For example, in man touch receptors in the skin of the trunk are connected by afferent fibres to interneurons at synapses in the dorsal horn of the spinal cord

HUMAN VISUAL PATHWAY

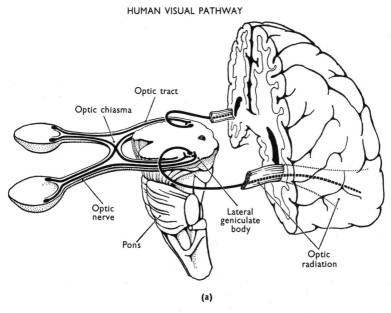

**Optic tract**

**Optic chiasma**

**Optic nerve**

**Pons**

**Lateral geniculate body**

**Optic radiation**

**(a)**

**Fig. 6–11**   (a) Scheme of visual pathway from retina to visual area of the human brain and (b) scheme of light reflex pathway (from retina, through midbrain, to sphincteric muscle of iris) and somatic reflex pathway. Afferent fibres which carry information concerned with the recognition of the object 'seen' by the eye end in the lateral geniculate body which is situated at the back of the brain stem and is part of the thalamic complex. Axons which form the optic radiation then sweep backwards to the visual area of the cortex. (From BASMAJIAN, 1964.)

(Fig. 6–7). These interneurons (sometimes called second sensory neurons) then usually, but not invariably, cross to the other side of the spinal cord and run up in the white matter of the cord to the brain in the lateral spino-thalamic tract. When they reach the brain they synapse with a second group of interneurons (third sensory neurons), in the thalamus which is a lower sensory centre. The third sensory neurons connect the thalamus with a higher sensory centre in the cerebral cortex.

Motor commands to muscles of the trunk and limbs from the higher motor centres in the cerebral cortex of man first travel along interneurons (upper motor neurons) to the medulla oblongata. At this point, most of the axons of the upper motor neurons cross to the other side of the central nervous system and continue down the spinal cord in the lateral cortico-spinal tract, while the rest pass down the cord in the anterior cortico-spinal tract (Fig. 6–10). The interneurons eventually synapse with motor neurons in the ventral (anterior) horn of the spinal cord. Since reflex activation of the body musculature is possible in a brainless animal, the complex connection between the brain and the spinal cord may seem rather unnecessary at first sight. However, even the simplest muscular activity requires very complex nervous integration for its smooth coordinated performance and once the influence of the brain is removed the ability to carry out movements in a smooth and effortless way is greatly impaired. Reflex movements, which are not controlled by the brain, do occur of course. These spinal reflexes are of great value for the performance of emergency activities such as movement of a finger away from a hot object. The brain is informed of the activity, but the information arrives too late for it to be actively involved in the execution of the act of withdrawal of the finger, although other responses of a somewhat less predictable and maybe unpublishable nature may follow this act!

Direct involvement of the brain occurs during reflex control of the mammalian eye. The visual pathways from the retina of the eye to the visual areas of the brain are illustrated in Fig. 6–11a. Afferent fibres which give a quantitative measure of the light entering the eye, reach the brain stem via the optic nerve and synapse with neurons situated in the transition zone between thalamus and midbrain (pretectal region). These, in turn, synapse with preganglionic parasympathetic neurons which send fibres along the oculomotor nerve to the ciliary ganglion just behind the eyeball. Postganglionic fibres then pass along the ciliary nerves to the iris muscles, which are responsible for controlling the pupil aperture, and to muscles which control the convexity of the lens so that objects may be accurately focused on the retina. By means of light reflexes the mammalian eye can make adjustments of the eye mechanism, according to the intensity of the light and the distance of an object from the eye (Fig. 6–11b). It can also initiate movements of the head or eyeballs by way of somatic reflexes (Fig. 6–11b).

To *some* extent, the behaviour of even the most complex animals is

## HUMAN LIGHT REFLEX PATHWAY

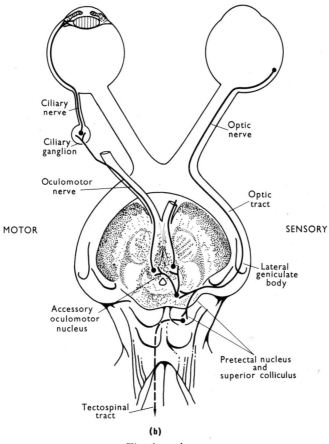

Fig. 6—11b

founded upon reflexes controlled by higher nervous centres. Indeed the most effective integration of sensory information can be achieved if this information can be brought into a single centre and then into contact with the motor units of the nervous system. Parts of the human brain are involved in collecting together and interpreting sensory inputs and it is here that our sensations are located. Information arriving in the central nervous system from most sensory receptors is in the form of action potentials and although in this form it may adequately describe the stimulus parameters, it does not define the stimulus modality. This can only be achieved through recognition by higher nervous centres of specific afferent pathways. The presence of such centres in the human brain is clearly indicated by the following experiment. If, for example, afferent fibres from a tactile receptor and an auditory receptor are severed and then rejoined so that the pathways are crossed, the input from the tactile receptor will now be interpreted as sound information, whereas that from the auditory receptor will be recognized as tactile information. In man the major sensory recognition areas of the brain are located within the cerebral

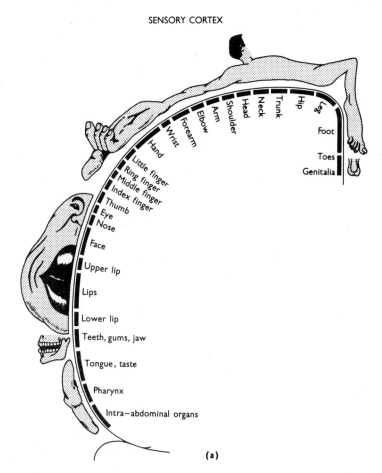

SENSORY CORTEX

(a)

**Fig. 6–12** The localization of function in (a) the somatic sensory cortex of man and (b) the motor cortex. Note the large areas devoted to sensation from and motor control of hands and face. Note also that the body is represented upside down although the face is not, itself, inverted. Each cerebral hemisphere controls the muscles on the contralateral side of the body. (After PENFIELD & RASMUSSEN, 1950.)

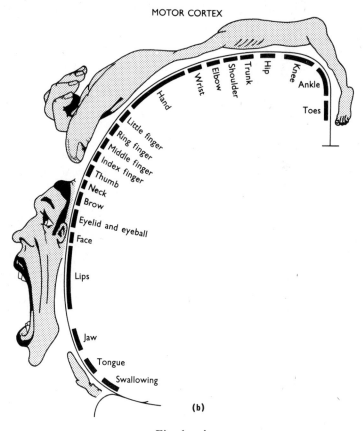

MOTOR CORTEX

**(b)**

Fig. 6–12b

cortex. This part of the brain also contains centres for generating command messages for controlling the body musculature. The sensory and motor areas of the cortex can be subdivided into smaller areas either monitoring or controlling specific activities of parts of the body (Fig. 6–12).

Complex stereotyped behaviour patterns are frequently initiated spontaneously within most nervous systems, in the absence of sensory influences, suggesting that these structures contain set programmes of activity. Even in animals, such as coelenterates, which do not have central nervous systems and well developed brains, behaviour cannot be completely described in terms of reflexes. It is clear that many behavioural activities are determined by preset nervous programmes producing fixed patterns of motor impulses. The regular opening and closing of the spiracles and the flight behaviour of some insects are examples of activities which are mainly centrally programmed. In vertebrates central programming of some forms of motor activity does occur, but most motor acts involve some reflex control. For example, the respiratory neurons in mammals which regulate diaphragm movements during breathing are programmed centrally and the activity of these neurons is not dependent on information from phasic sensory receptors monitoring the breathing apparatus although the respiratory pattern may be regulated in terms of its repetition frequency by information from tonic sensory receptors. The physiological mechanisms underlying centrally programmed activities are not well understood although spontaneously active central neurons or groups of neurons are usually involved. These neurons usually have very unstable membrane potentials which drift slowly towards the critical depolarization threshold. On reaching the depolarization threshold an action potential is generated. After repolarization the membrane potential slowly drifts once again towards threshold. The cardiac ganglia found on the hearts of crustaceans such as lobsters and crabs, contain nine to fifteen spontaneously active neurons which interact to initiate bursts of impulses which excite the heart. This integrative process maintains the heartbeat in these animals, and possibly reflects the sort of neuronal interaction responsible for the production of patterns of nerve impulses associated with more complex behavioural activities in these and other animals.

# Memory

Experiential information greatly influences the behaviour of most animals and it is generally assumed that memories or records of past experiences, which enable animals to relate what is happening now with previous experiences, are stored in nervous systems. At least superficially, therefore, a nervous system is like a computer since it receives information, processes information and has a memory store. However, it is somewhat misleading to carry this analogy too far. For example, modern digital computers consist in the main of binary units or two-way switches each of which can handle no more than two simultaneous signals whereas neurons may be simultaneously influenced by several hundred other nerve cells. Furthermore, a computer can usually only handle information that has first been carefully processed by the operator whereas a nervous system does its own processing and is able to sort out relevant data from irrelevant data. Although the human brain works about one million times slower than a computer it is nevertheless able to perform many different operations simultaneously and also appears to have more ready access to its memory since it does not have to sift systematically through its bank of information. A nervous system is also less likely to break down because many neurons perform the same task. This redundancy ensures that loss of some neurons does not markedly influence overall performance. In a computer each unit performs a specific function and when one unit fails the results are often quite catastrophic.

A hypothetical scheme for memory storage in the optic lobe of the octopus brain based upon two-way switches has been proposed, the binary units being called mnemons. A diagrammatic presentation of one of these memory units is illustrated in Fig. 7-1. Visual information received by the dendrites of the classifying cell is passed on to motor cells, which cause either attack or retreat of the animal, according to their 'resting' state. It is assumed that initially the unit will be biased towards the attack mode. If attack occurs and it is rewarded by food capture, then taste receptors in the mouth will reinforce the output of the attack motor cell. At the same time, the output from the attack motor cell will, through a collateral pathway involving a memory cell, inhibit any activity of the retreat motor cell. If, however, attack is not rewarded by food capture but is followed instead by a pain stimulus, e.g. an electric shock, the retreat motor cell will be activated and the attack motor cell inhibited. Many thousands of these binary units would be involved in controlling the behaviour of the octopus, the behaviour at any one time depending on the number of units switched for attack compared to the number switched for retreat. It is possible to train the octopus to associate food and pain

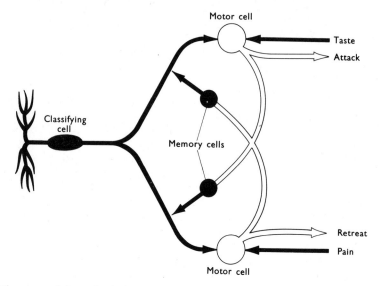

**Fig. 7–1** A hypothetical memory unit (mnemon) in the optic lobe of the octopus.

with certain objects, presumably as a result of the specific arrangement of the classifying cells and their dendritic process in the optic lobe of this mollusc, different objects exciting different groups of classifying cells. Learning in this animal therefore appears to be a choice between two alternatives and the learning process involves closing one of the channels of the mnemon by means of the collateral inhibitory pathways. If these changes are to persist for more than a few seconds, the memory cells must be capable of having some long-term effect on the output of the motor cells. There is no evidence, as yet, that inhibitory synaptic pathways can have long-term effects of the type envisaged in this model, although any synaptic changes that do occur as a result of exciting one of the collateral inhibitory pathways, could presumably be reinforced by repetition. If such long-term synaptic effects do occur, then the problem of erasure of the memory trace is raised. Once the octopus has come to associate a particular shape with food, how are the mnemons, associated with that shape, switched to the retreat mode if that shape becomes associated with pain? Undoubtedly they could be completely inactivated by exciting the inhibitory pathway to the attack motor cell, but some method for disinhibiting the retreat motor cell would also be necessary for complete resetting of the system to take account of the new situation.

Although computer-like models of the mnemon type play a valuable role in our investigations of the complexities of nervous organization they usually grossly oversimplify the situation, being all too frequently based on insufficient structural and physiological information. However, macro-molecular and perhaps also behavioural studies of experiential information storage in nervous systems are not quite so handicapped in this respect, and it seems worth while to consider these in some detail.

## 7.1   Short-term memory in insects

It has been suggested that nervous systems store information in two different ways. Information that is stored for anything from a few minutes to a few days is said to constitute short-term memory whereas information that is stored for longer periods constitutes long-term memory. A simple experiment can be performed to demonstrate short-term memory in insects (Fig. 7–2). A headless cockroach or locust is suspended above a dish of saline, so that when the insect extends its metathoracic leg (prothoracic or mesothoracic legs can equally well be used), the tarsal segments enter the fluid. The end of a piece of fine wire is wrapped around the tibial segment and connected to one side of a stimulator (an electronic device that gives brief electric shocks; see Studies in Biology no. 11).

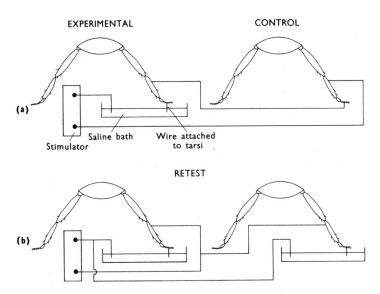

**Fig. 7–2** Diagram of circuits for investigating short-term memory in insects. (a) Training circuit used to condition either a cockroach or a locust to avoid an electric shock. When the circuit is completed by the experimental animal as it dips its foot into the saline, both the experimental and control animals are shocked. (b) Retest circuits. Both the experimental and control animals are treated in the same way. See text for further explanation. (After HORRIDGE, 1962.)

The other side of the stimulator is connected to the saline bath so that when the leg enters the saline it completes the circuit and the animal receives a series of shocks from the stimulator (at a stimulus frequency of 1 stimulus 1 sec). A second insect, which acts as a control, is wired in series with the experimental animal and is shocked each time the experimental animal is shocked regardless of the position of the metathoracic leg of the control animal. The experimental animal 'learns' within about 10 min to keep its leg out of the saline, whereas the control animal does not 'learn' to raise its leg, even though both animals receive the same number of shocks. It appears that the experimental animal 'learns' to relate the position of its metathoracic leg to the presence or absence of the stimulus and to regulate leg position in order to avoid stimulation. After the experimental animal has been trained for about 1 hour, it is then rested for 10 min before the experiment is repeated (retest, Fig. 7-2b). This time, however, the control animal is treated in exactly the same way as the experimental animal. By this means, it is possible to demonstrate that the experimental animal has remembered its previous training and receives significantly less shocks than the control animal (Fig. 7-3). By studying the activity of motor neurons to the muscles in the locust leg which are responsible for leg raising, it has been

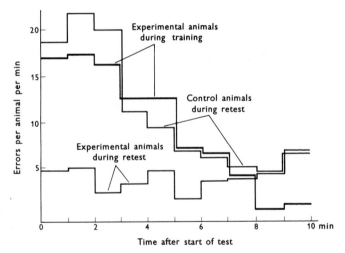

**Fig. 7-3** Results from an experiment in which the right hind legs of two sets of locusts were trained as in Fig. 7-2 (a) and then retested as in Fig. 7-2 (b). The number of shocks for twenty experimental and twenty control animals are plotted for each minute interval following the start of the retest. Note that the experimental animals receive far fewer shocks than the control animals. The number of shocks received by the experimental animals when first trained are indicated by the thick lines and the trend is seen to be similar to that shown by the control animals during the retest. (After HORRIDGE, 1962.)

possible to gain some insight into the changes in output from the central nervous system which accompany leg raising behaviour in this insect. For example, one of these muscles, namely the metathoracic anterior coxal adductor muscle, is innervated by a motor neuron which fires more or less continuously. When the afferent fibres in the metathoracic leg are shocked and the shocks are timed to follow significant falls in the firing frequency of this motor neuron, a transitory rise in impulse frequency occurs. Further selectively timed stimuli produce further increases in the firing frequency, which are maintained for progressively longer periods. It is also possible to lower the firing frequency of the motor neuron by timing shocks to occur following spontaneous bursts of action potentials at frequencies higher than average. Apparently stimulation of leg afferents reverses ongoing activity so that leg-lowering becomes leg-raising, an increase in impulse frequency becomes a decrease in impulse frequency and a decrease in impulse frequency reverts to an increase. There is little doubt that changes occur in the metathoracic ganglion of the central nervous system of these insects during the training procedure, possibly at the level of the synaptic contacts between afferent and efferent neurons, although interneurons may also be involved. But the effects of training are not restricted to the metathoracic segment, since it can be shown that prothoracic and mesothoracic legs learn to avoid shocks more quickly if a metathoracic leg has been trained to do so. This, of course, reflects the extensiveness of the neuronal coupling between segments in insects.

## 7.2　Synapses and short-term memory

One obvious site for storage of short-term memory is the synapse. Facilitation at excitatory and inhibitory synapses and synaptic fatigue could account for short-term memories which are retained for a few minutes. For example, imagine a motor neuron with inputs from five different afferent neurons. Normally an impulse in any one of these afferents is insufficient to depolarize the motor neuron beyond its threshold for spike generation. To do this it is necessary to excite all five afferents more or less simultaneously. However, if one afferent is stimulated repetitively synaptic facilitation results eventually in the appearance of a spike in the motor neuron. For as long as this facilitation lasts, this single input will be capable of activating the motor neuron. Information has been stored in the facilitated synapse which takes cognizance of its previous history and has changed its effectiveness or weighting with respect to the other synapses. Apart from changes in synaptic weighting, other possible ways of storing information at synapses include saturation of the mechanism, which absorbs the transmitters or their products from synaptic clefts, and depletion of enzymes responsible for either degrading synaptic transmitters or for limiting the time course of the interaction between transmitter and postsynaptic receptor. Indeed, there is evidence that at cholinergic synapses in the central nervous system of the cockroach either a fall in cholinesterase level or a change in conformation of the cholinesterase to a less active state is involved in the changes in leg raising behaviour referred to earlier. On the postsynaptic side, changes in the electrical properties of the non-synaptic neuron membrane may occur during repeated stimulation of the cell. Mechanisms which could account for short-term memories, which are retained for hours rather than minutes, are less easy to imagine, but may conceivably be similar to those described above. An alternative idea is that all short-term memories are stored in neuron circuits, so-called reverberatory circuits, as travelling waves of electricity, i.e. action potentials. Although there is little evidence to support this idea, it does have interesting possibilities, since information stored in circuits of this type could be played over and over again to produce changes which eventually constitute long-term memory, without the need for repetition of the experiences.

### 7.3   Long-term memory

There are two main lines of thought concerning long-term memory. On the one hand, it has been suggested that experimental information is stored in nervous systems over long periods of time as macromolecules, in much the same way that genetic information is stored. On the other hand, long-term memory is believed to have a structured basis and to involve changes in structure and therefore properties of neurons.

### 7.4   DNA, RNA and memory

The complex stereotyped behavioural patterns of some animals provide the most dramatic evidence that information deriving from parental deoxyribonucleic acid (DNA) defines and activates the neuronal networks appropriate to the behavioural patterns. This process presumably depends upon ribonucleic acids (RNA) acting as messengers which read-out the DNA-encoded instructions and that dictate and stabilize the neuronal junctions required for stereotyped behaviour. Because the genome contains information on behaviour of this type and because of the major role of DNA in encoding genetic information in general, it has been proposed that this macromolecule could also encode experiential information. However, DNA is a very stable molecule and unlikely to undergo the sort of chemical alterations that would be responsible for continuous memory storage.

The case for RNA as a memory molecule is somewhat more compelling. It has been reported that when RNA is extracted from trained flatworms (*Planaria*) and fed to untrained 'worms' the effects of training can be transferred from the trained to the naïve subjects. Similar results have been obtained by injecting untrained rats or mice with RNA from brains of trained animals. However, when the mouse brain is given actinomycin D, an antibiotic which inhibits RNA synthesis, learning is not abolished. Unfortunately, the results of experiments of this type are difficult to evaluate and have, in the past, been subjected to considerable adverse critical comment. There is a lot of evidence that moderate nervous activity leads to an increase of up to 100% in the RNA content of the active neurons. However, the RNA content of most cells increases with activity, so this does not necessarily directly implicate RNA in nervous information storage. Nevertheless, increases in RNA content of active neurons suggest that the protein synthesis capacity of these cells also increases. Many studies have been made to determine the effects of nervous activity and inactivity on the rate of synthesis and degradation of brain proteins, some of the most elegant involving goldfish. For example, when a goldfish is placed in a shuttlebox it readily learns to leap over a 'fence' from one chamber to the other chamber to avoid a repeated electrical shock which is preceded by a warning light, and it retains this ability for days after the training period. Puromycin interferes with the retention of the learnt behaviour, although it has no effect on learning during the training period. It appears, therefore, to block long-term memory whilst leaving short-term memory unimpaired. Long-term memory is most effectively blocked if puromycin is applied for up to 60 minutes after training, which suggests that the memory trace is established by this time. Since long-term memory fixation in goldfish can also be blocked by actinomycin D, it appears that both RNA synthesis and protein synthesis are involved in this process. There is, however, need for some caution in interpreting the results of protein inhibition studies in connection with memory. For example, if puromycin is injected intracranially into mice after training in a maze, information about the maze cannot be recalled. It seems reasonable to assume from this that the puromycin has blocked long-term memory formation. However, information about the maze can be readily recalled even two months after training, simply by injecting physiological saline intracranially into puromycin treated mice. It seems, therefore, that in this instance puromycin had not prevented long-term memory fixation, but had merely prevented the recall of stored information. Possibly this substance blocks neural pathways by preventing transmitter release from nerve terminals, the effect of the saline being to flush the puromycin from these sites.

If it is accepted that memory fixation is dependent upon synthesis of new proteins which are presumably used for modifying neuronal structure and function, then there is the problem of how these protein products are disseminated throughout the neuron, particularly if the neuron has a long axon. The major production site of neuronal constituents and the area of their consumption are not intermingled and coextensive, but rather neatly compartmentalized, most of the protein, for example, being manufactured in the soma. Unlike the soma and dendrites, the axon is devoid of Nissl granules and contains scattered ribosomes only in the initial segment (Fig. 1–2). Thus the axon proper, which can attain a volume one thousand times as large as the soma volume, is apparently free of ribosomes, the organelles known to be required for protein synthesis. Some local axonal synthesis of proteins does occur especially by mitochondria, although usually for their own needs. Nevertheless, the fact that mitochondria are concentrated in axon terminals (Plate 5), indicates that at these sites some of the protein manufactured by these organelles may be used for other purposes. Possibly carbohydrates are added to preformed polypeptides at axon terminals to form glycoproteins, substances which could play an important role in modifying the surface of the terminals and therefore transmitter release. The glial cells which accompany axons may also provide some additional protein. This is suggested by the remarkable observation that crustacean motor axons can survive for many months when separated from their somata.

The need to transport proteins manufactured in the soma to distant axonal sites necessitates an organized traffic system. This is provided by axoplasmic flow up and down axons at rates between about 0·25 mm/day and 100 cm/day. It seems possible that fast axoplasmic flow involves the neurotubules which are aligned longitudinally in the axon, since when these structures are disrupted by colchicine, this form of axoplasmic flow stops. The concept of axoplasmic flow has emerged from observations that surplus axoplasm piles up at the proximal side of a chronic nerve constriction, whilst there is a reduction in axoplasm accompanied by a corresponding reduction in fibre diameter at the distal side. Undoubtedly axoplasmic flow is involved in causing these changes, although the 'pile-up' phenomenon results mainly from *axon* flow. An axon constantly moves in a proximal-distal direction away from its soma and this process leads to $10^4$ internal self-renewals of an axon during the lifetime of a neuron. This staggering observation is a convincing indication of the plasticity of the nerve cell. Axon flow, like axoplasmic flow, might, therefore, play an important role in storage of experiential information.

## 7.5 Synapses and long-term memory

Regions of the vertebrate nervous system that are implicated in the ready storage of information are characterized by having layers of profoundly overlapping dendritic trees from somata in other layers, with glial cells interspersed among the dendrites. Such a structure is characteristic of the mammalian cortex and it is a phyletic difference in that the more advanced the animal the greater the volume of dendrites in proportion to somata. It has often been assumed, therefore, that there is a relationship between dendritic volume and capacity of the memory bank. Since the dendrites are of prime importance for synaptic function, it is not surprising that they have been extensively studied by those interested in transfer and storage of nervous information. Recently the dendritic spine has been under the spotlight. The dendritic spine was discovered about 60 years ago and has, for a long time, been considered of value in increasing the dendritic area for synaptic contact with other neurons. However, since many dendrites with these spines have extensive synapse-free areas this argument appears to be somewhat untenable. Indeed synaptic contacts on mammalian motor neurons are almost exclusively limited to the dendritic spines. It has recently been suggested that the dendritic spine forms a postsynaptic region which is effectively isolated from other synapses on the neuron so that its activity is not influenced by the present or past behaviour of these other synapses. This means that if transmission at any one spine synapse becomes more effective through usage then its contribution to the final output of the dendrite and postsynaptic neuron (in other words, its synaptic weighting) will correspondingly increase. Another suggestion is that the base of the spine may increase in diameter with usage and that this would result in less attenuation of the synaptic potential as it spread electronically from the spine into the dendrite. Although these ideas are rather speculative, changes in structure and function of dendritic spines could be involved in the laying down of a memory trace. The possibility that presynaptic nerve terminals migrate up and down the postsynaptic cell or that new synaptic connections are formed during learning must also be considered. It has been recently demonstrated that, with repeated usage, the terminals of some presynaptic neurons in the vertebrate brain increase in size and that their area of contact with their postsynaptic counterparts increases. This could increase synaptic efficacy and might be one method of information storage.

## 7.6 Memory in mammals

Mammals have both long- and short-term memories. When humans are given certain types of electric shock therapy, they usually have no recollection of the events in the half-hour period preceding the treatment and when other mammals such as rats are trained to perform a specific task, they forget their training, if their brains are given a powerful electric shock a few minutes after the training session. However, electric shocks are incapable of erasing mammalian memory once it has become established for about an hour or so.

The hippocampus and temporal lobes of the cerebral cortex play a major role in establishing long-term memory traces or engrams in man. When these structures are removed new memories cannot be established. However, they are not the storage sites for long-term memories since their removal does not prevent the recall of past experiential information.

Memory traces appear to be distributed throughout the human brain but removal of part of the brain tissue does not, as one might expect, remove some memories completely, although details of memory traces are lost, their overall pattern is not greatly affected. It seems likely, therefore, that the memory traces are either very diffusely distributed or multiplicated and established in many parts of the brain. This does not mean, of course, that all brain neurons and all brain synapses are involved in long-term information storage. Some neurons are not labile and so do not change their properties with usage. These stable cells perform tasks that are determined before the nervous system develops and which remain constant throughout the life of the animal. Many of the neurons involved in important activities like vision and respiration come into this category and could be considered to constitute a pool of nerve cells containing hereditable or genetic memory.

Most of man's brain is concerned with analysing afferent information in relation to previous experience, sensory and motor. The mechanism of human thought depends on correlating one memory with another. This process does not appear to be dependent upon the possession of any special type of cell in the brain but rather on the fact that man has a larger number of neurons and a greater capacity for developing complicated inter-neuron connections than other animals.

A lot of progress will be made during the next decade in understanding the physiological basis and structural basis for storage of experiential information in nervous systems and in understanding the molecular basis for the electrical phenomena which occur in nerve cells. Scientists with markedly different backgrounds will be involved in this exciting venture and maybe eventually we shall even know all there is to know about that enigmatic structure, the human brain.

# Books for further reading

CASE, J. (1966). *Sensory Mechanisms.* The Macmillan Company, London and New York.
GUROWITZ, E. M. (1969). *The Molecular Basis of Memory.* Prentice-Hall, Inc., Englewood Cliffs, New Jersey.
MCLENNAN, H. (1963). *Synaptic Transmission.* W. B. Saunders and Company, Philadelphia.
VAN DER KLOOT, W. G. (1968). *Behaviour.* Holt, Rinehart and Winston, Inc., New York and London.
WILKIE, D. R. (1968). *Muscle.* Studies in Biology, No. 11, Edward Arnold, London.
YOUNG, J. Z. (1964). *A Model of the Brain.* Oxford University Press, Oxford.

# References

Books indicated * are recommended for further reading.

ALBRECHT, F. O. (1953). *The Anatomy of the Migratory Locust.* The Athlone Press, London
BASMAJIAN, J. V. (1964). *Primary Anatomy,* Williams and Wilkins. Baltimore
BUCHSBAUM, R. (1948). *Animals without Backbones.* University of Chicago Press, Chicago
*BULLOCK, T. A. and HORRIDGE, G. A. (1965). *Structure and Function in the Nervous System of Invertebrates.* 1. Freeman, London and San Francisco
GRAY, E. G. (1960). The fine structure of the insect ear. *Phil. Trans. B.,* **203,** 75
*GREGORY, R. L. (1966). *Eye and Brain.* Weidenfeld and Nicolson, London
HARDY, M. (1935). Observations on the innervation of the macula sacculi in man. *Anat. Rec.,* **59,** 403
HODGKIN, A. L. and HUXLEY, A. F. (1952). A quantitative description of membrane current and its application to conduction and excitation in nerve. *J. Physiol.,* **117,** 500
HODGKIN, A. L. and KEYNES, R. D. (1955). Active transport of cations into giant axons from *Sepia* and *Loligo, J. Physiol.,* **128,** 28
HORRIDGE, G. A. (1962). Learning of leg position by the ventral nerve cord in headless insects. *Proc. R. Soc. B.,* **157,** 33
*HORRIDGE, G. A. (1968). *Interneurons. Their Origin, Action, Specificity Growth and Plasticity.* W. H. Freeman, London and San Francisco
*HUBBARD, J. I., LLINAS, R. and QUASTEL, D. M. J. (1969). *Electrophysiological Analysis of Synaptic Transmission.* Edward Arnold, London
JOSEPHSON, R. (1961). Colonial responses of hydroid polyps. *J. exp. Biol.,* **38,** 559

118 REFERENCES

*KATZ, B. (1966). *Nerve, Muscle and Synapse.* McGraw-Hill, New York and London

KRAVITZ, E. A., MOLINOFF, P. B. and HALL, Z. W. (1965). A comparison of the enzymes and substrates of γ-aminobutyric acid metabolism in lobster excitatory and inhibitory axons. *Proc. Nat. Acad. Sci. U.S.A.,* **54,** 778

MAXIMOV, A. A. and BLOOM, W. (1957). *Textbook of Histology.* W. B. Saunders, Philadelphia

*McNAUGHT, A. B. and CALLANDER, R. (1970). *Illustrated Physiology.* E. and S. Livingstone, Edinburgh and London

NAKAJIMA, S. and ONODERA, K. (1969). Membrane properties of the stretch receptor neurone of crayfish with particular reference to mechanism of sensory adaptation. *J. Physiol.,* **200,** 191

PARKER, T. J. and HASWELL, W. A. (1951). *A Text-book of Zoology,* II. Macmillan, London

PENFIELD, W. G. and RASMUSSEN, T. (1950). *The Cerebral Cortex of Man.* Macmillan, London and New York

SÉGUY, E. (1951). Ordre des Diptères. In *Grassé's Traité de Zoologie,* **10,** 449. Masson & Cie, Paris

SHIPLEY, A. E. and MACBRIDE, E. W. (1920). *Zoology, an Elementary Text-book.* Cambridge University Press, London

SHOLL, D. A. (1956). *The Organization of the Cerebral Cortex.* Methuen and Company Ltd., London; John Wiley, New York

SNODGRASS, R. E. (1935). *Principles of Insect Morphology.* McGraw-Hill, London

USHERWOOD, P. N. R. (1967). Insect neuromuscular mechanisms. *Am. Zool.,* **7,** 553

UVAROV, B. (1966). *Grasshoppers and Locusts.* Cambridge University Press, London

VON FRISCH, K. (1936). Über der Gehörsinn der Fische. *Biol. Rev.,* **11,** 210

WELSH, J. H., SMITH, R. I. and KAMMER, A. (1968). *Laboratory Exercises in Invertebrate Physiology.* Burgess, Minneapolis

WIGGLESWORTH, V. B. (1965). *The Principles of Insect Physiology.* Methuen, London

WOOD, D. W. (1968). *Animal Physiology.* Edward Arnold, London

WYBURN, G. M., PICKFORD, R. W. and HIRST, R. J. (1964). *Human Senses and Perception.* University of Toronto Press, Toronto

YOUNG, J. Z. (1967). Neural networks. *Science Journal,* **3,** 52.

# Index

Italics indicate pages containing one or more relevant text-figures.

Acetylcholine  *54–9*
Adaptation  *62–4*, 93, 99
Adenosinetriphosphate (ATP)  *34–5*
γ-Aminobutyrate  *54–5*
Amphibian
  Frog  19, *48–9*, 54, 56–7, 59, *72–3*, Plate 6
  Toad  *72–3*
Annelid  13, 83
  Earthworm  21
Arthropod  *2*, *4*, *13–14*, 24, 54, *56–9*, 66, 79, *81*, 93, 96
Axon (nerve fibre)  2–9, 13, 17, 42, 48, *52–4*, 92, 113–14, Plates 2, 3
  Afferent (sensory)  9, 19, 24, 64, *76*, 81, 85, *96*, 99, 111
  Efferent (motor)  9, 19, 24, *100–2*, 114
  Flow  114
  Giant  *35*, *46–7*
  Hillock  *3*, 91–2
  Myelinated  4, *23*, *45–7*, Plates 2, 3
  Non-myelinated  23, *45–6*, Plates 2, 3
Axoplasm  42, 46, 114
  Flow  114

Basilar membrane  *70*, 72
Bird  21, 72, 74
  Owl  84
Bouton  *3*
Brain  5, *12–15*, 18, 72, 81, 83–6, 97–105, 115–16
  Lamprey  *20*
  Locust  *14*
  Horse  *20*
  Human  *16*, *100–5*
  Vertebrate  *16–21*

Cerebellum  *20–1*

Cerebral cortex  *2*, 5, 21, *98*, *100–5*, 114–15, Plate 1
Cerebral hemispheres  19–21, 104
Cholinesterase  59, 112
Cochlea  *68–70*, 72
Coelenterate  *2*, *4*, *7–12*, 83, 93, 96, 105
  Coral  10, 93
  *Hydra*  10
  Jellyfish (*Aurelia*)  *10–12*, *94*
  Sea Anemone  10, 12
Conduction
  Axonal  *42–9*
  Saltatory  49
  Velocity  46–7, 49, *94*
Cornea  *81*, 83
Crustacean  4, 55, 60, *65–6*, 77, 80, 86, 98, 114
  Crab  86–7, 106
  Crayfish  *63–4*, *76*, 78
  Lobster  *65*, 76, 80, 99, 106
Crystalline cone  *79–81*
Crystalline tract  *79–81*

Depolarization  38, *42–7*, *52–4*, 56, 58–60, *62–4*, *88*
Dendrite  *2–6*, 42, *61–2*, 66, 75, 91–2, 99, 107–8, 114
Dendritic spine  *2*, *6*, 115
DNA  112
Donnan equilibrium  30, 34

Ear
  Drum *see* Membrane, tympanic
  External  66
  Internal (inner)  *66–8*, *72–3*
  Middle  *66–8*, *72–3*
  Ossicles  *see* Malleus, incus, stapes
Echinoderm  12

Effector   1, 5, 7–9, 13, 18, 22, 24, 52, 61
Electrode   25–7, 43–51
   Anode   25–7, 43, 44
   Cathode   25–7, 43–51
Electrolyte   25–7, 30
Eustachian tube   67–8
Eye   1, 3, 14, 61, 76, 79–87
   Compound   79–84, Plates 7, 8
   Mammalian   84, 102
   Simple   see Ocellus
   Vertebrate   83–7

Facet   79–81, Plate 8
Facilitation   88, 111
Fish   19, 21, 72–3, 77, 113
   Goldfish   1, 60, 113
   Lamprey   20
   Myxine   16

Ganglion   9, 10–15, 17, 22–4, 102, 106, Plate 4
Glial cell   18, 114, Plates 2–3

Helicotrema   68
Hyperpolarization   42, 44, 58, 60, 64
Hypothalamus   19

Incus   67–8
Inhibition
   Central   101
   Peripheral   55, 93
   Presynaptic   60, 90, 92–3
   Postsynaptic   90–3
Innervation
   Multiterminal   56–7, 93
   Polyneuronal   57, 93
   Reciprocal   96, 101
Insect   4, 13, 74, 79–80, 86, 97, 105, 109–11
   Cockroach   14, 109, 112
   Fly   14–15, 86, Plate 8
   Lacewing   74

Locust   14, 49, 74–5, 82, 86–7, 109–11, Plates 5, 8, 9
Moth   74, 80
Internode   4–5, 48
Ion
   Anion   25–31, 34
   Calcium   52, 54
   Cation   25–31, 34
   Chloride   25–31, 34, 36, 56, 58, 62, 64
   Mobility   28, 30
   Potassium   30, 31, 34–6, 42, 56, 58, 62, 64
   Sodium   25–42, 45, 56, 62, 64
   Sulphate   30–1
Iris   83–4

Labyrinth
   Bony   68
   Membranous   68–72, 77
Lagena   72–4, 77
Lens   79, 81, 83–5, 102

Malleus   67–8
Mammal   5, 19. 21, 64, 70, 72, 98, 101, 106, 115
   Bat   74
   Cat   2, Plate 1
   Dolphin   74
   Man   9–10, 66, 68, 73, 79, 83–5, 96–7, 116
   Mouse   112–13
   Rabbit   1
   Rat   112, 115, Plate 3
Medulla oblongata   21, 98, 102
Membrane
   Artificial   30–2, 34
   Axon   46–8
   Dendrite   3, 62
   Neuron   25, 32–4, 37, 38, 40–2, 45, 49, 112
   Non-synaptic   56–9, 93, 112
   Presynaptic   6–7, 52–5, 59–60, Plate 5
   Postsynaptic   6–7, 53–60, Plate 5
   Soma   3

Memory   1, 87, 107–11, 115
  Long-term   112–16
  Molecule   112
  Short-term   109–13   115
  Trace (Engram)   108, 115–16
Mitochondria   3, 6, 114, Plate 5
Mnemon   107–8
Mollusc   14–15, 59
  Cuttlefish (Sepia)   35
  Octopus   15–16, 107–9
  Snail   Plate 4
Muscle   1, 6–9, 12, 14, 18–19, 21–2,
    24, 54–60, 65–7, 83–4, 88,
    93–4, 96, 98–106, 111, Plate 5
  Spindle   18, 67, 96
Myelin   4–5, 17, 45, 47–9, Plate 2, 3


Nerve   4
  Cord   13, 15
  Cranial   16–19, 23–4
  Net   8, 10–13, 93–5
  Plexus   12–15
  Ring   12
  Spinal   16–19, 100
Neurohormone   4, 7, 24
Neuron   2, Plate 1
  Amacrine   3, 84
  Cholinergic   54–5
  Excitatory   57, 66, 93, 99
  Inhibitory   54–5, 57,   60, 66, 93,
    99
  Inter-   6, 8–9, 17–18, 97–105, 111
  Mauthner   21, 60
  Motor (efferent)   2, 8–9, 17–18,
    54, 56–7, 59, 67, 93, 96–7, 99–
    102, 111, 115, Plate 5
  Parasympathetic   22–4, 54, 102
  Sensory (afferent)   2, 9, 17–18,
    51–4, 66–7, 75, 96–9, 101–2, 111
  Sympathetic   22–4
Neurotubule   3, 4, 54, 114
Node of Ranvier   4–5, 45, 47–8


Ocellus   82–3
Ommatidium   79–81, Plate 8
Optic lobe   21, 81, 107–8
Optic nerve   16, 21, 101–2

Optokinesis   86–7, Plate 9
Organ of Corti   70
Otolith   79
Oval window (Fenestra ovalis)   67–8,
    70, 73


Permeability   30–40, 53, 57–8, 62,
    64
  Chloride   41, 62
  Potassium   38–42, 58, 62
  Sodium   38–41, 58, 62
Pigment
  Cell   79–81
  Photochemical (visual)   81, 85–6
Platyhelminth   (flatworm)   12–14,
    49, 83
  Planaria   13, 112
Pons   21
Potential
  Action   3, 37–41, 42–60, 62–3, 76,
    81, 88–95, 103, 106, 111–12
  After-   40
  Chloride equilibrium   58–9
  Diffusion   28–30
  Electrotonic   42–4
  Generator   37, 64
  Potassium equilibrium   30,   36,
    40, 56, 58–9
  Receptor   37, 62–4, 81, 99
  Resting   34–7, 58–9
  Sodium equilibrium   39–40, 56
  Synaptic   see Synaptic potential
Pump
  Electrogenic   35, 59
  Potassium   34–5, 42
  Sodium   34–5, 40, 42, 59


Refractoriness   38, 44–6, 49–50, 93
Reissner's membrane   70
Reflex   17–18, 76, 78, 96–106
Repolarization   39, 43, 58, 106
Reptile   21, 72, 74
Retina   61, 79, 81, 83–5, 87, 101–2
Retinula cell   79–81
Rhabdom   79, 81
Rhopalium   10–11
RNA   112–13

Round window (Fenestra rotunda)
   68, 70


Sacculus   68, 70, 73, 77
Scala media   68, 70
Scala tympani   68, 70
Schwann cell   4-5, Plates 2, 3
Semicircular canals   68-70, 77
Sensory receptor   1, 5, 7-9, 12,
   61-88
   Auditory   61, 65-75, 104
   Chemo-   61
   Cone   61, 83-6
   Electro-   64
   Equilibrium   68, 70, 75-9
   Muscle   63, 65-6, 98
   Phasic   62, 64-5, 106
   Photo-   64, 79-86
   Pressure   98
   Rod   61, 83-6
   Stretch   63, 66, 98
   Taste   61, 107
   Tendon   67, 99
   Thermo-   64
   Tonic   62, 64-5, 106
   Touch (Tactile)   98, 101, 104
Spider   82
Spinal cord   8, 16-19, 21, 23, 96,
   98, 100-2
Stapes   67-8
Statocyst   75-8
Statolith   11, 76
Summation
   Temporal   88, 93
   Spatial   89-90, 93
Synapse   3, 5-7, 10, 13, 18, 24, 37,
   52-60, 88-102, 111-12, 115,
   Plates 4, 5
   Electrical   5, 7, 60
   Excitatory   53-6, 58, 60, 88-92,
   111
   Chemical   '5-7, 10, 52-60
   Cholinergic   55-8, 112
   Inhibitory   55, 58, 60, 85, 89,
   91-3, 108, 111
   Nerve-muscle   6-7, 56-8
Synaptic cleft   6-7, 10, 52-4, 59-60,
   111
Synaptic current   53, 56, 58, 60,
   91-2
Synaptic delay   54, 60
Synaptic fatigue   89, 93, 111
Synaptic potential   37, 58-9, 88-95,
   115
   Excitatory   58, 88-95
   Inhibitory   90-5
Synaptic receptor   53-60, 111
Synaptic vesicle   6-7, 52, 54, 58,
   Plate 5


Tapetum   84
Tectorial membrane   68, 70
Thalamus   19, 101-2
Threshold   38, 42, 44, 46, 49, 56,
   60, 106
Transmitter   4, 6-7, 52-6, 58-60,
   64, 111, 114
   Excitatory   52-8
   Inhibitory   54, 58
Tympanal organ   44-75
Tympanic membrane   66-8, 70-3,
   75